the low-carb
diet for life

linda gassenheimer

Kyle Cathie Limited

the low-carb
diet for life

By the author of *Low-Carb Meals in Minutes*

linda gassenheimer

Kyle Cathie Limited

To Harold for his love of good food and his enthusiastic support for this project.

First published in Great Britain 2003 by

Kyle Cathie Limited

122 Arlington Road

London NW1 7HP

www.kylecathie.com

general.enquiries@kyle-cathie.com

ISBN 1 85626 462 9

Text © 2003 Linda Gassenheimer

Project Editor: Helen Woodhall

Editorial Assistant: Esme West

Designer: Mark Buckingham

Special Photography and Styling: Juliet Piddington

Home Economy: Carol Tennant

Anglicisation: Nicole Foster

Production: Lorraine Baird and Sha Huxtable

Linda Gassenheimer is hereby identified as the author of this work in accordance with Section 77 of the Copyright, Designs and Patents Act 1988.

A Cataloguing In Publication record for this title is available from the British Library.

Colour separations by Scanhouse

Printed and bound by Kyodo

contents

Introduction 7
Special Features
Smart Shopping the Low-Carb Way
Shopping Guidelines
Staples
Equipment
Quick Cooking Tips and Helpful Hints
Tips for Eating Out
Quick Snacks

Quick Star 26
Breakfast
Mid-Morning Snack
Lunch
Mid-Afternoon Snack
Dinner
Quick Start 14-Day Meal Plan

Quick Start Breakfasts 30
Bacon and Cheese Crêpes
Microwave Eggs Parmesan
Mushroom, Turkey and Tarragon
  Omelette
Turkey Salsa Roll
Microwave Marinara Scramble
Smoked Salmon-Stuffed Celery
Sausage and Artichoke Frittata

Quick Start Lunches 38
Sicilian Baked Mushrooms and
  Sausage
Chicken with Dill Mustard
Cheese and Chicken Bundles
Nutty Chicken Minestrone
Spanish Tuna-Stuffed Tomatoes
Crunchy Oriental Chicken Salad
Crab Gratin

Quick Start Dinners 46
Hot Pepper Prawns
Mediterranean Baked Fish
Chicken Burgers with Warm
  Mushroom Salad
Crab Cakes and Slaw
Pork Escalopes with Spinach and
  Mushrooms
Roasted Salmon and Herb Sauce
Tuscan Chicken

Which Carbs 56
Breakfast
Lunch

Dinner
Which Carbs 14-Day Meal Plan

Which Carbs Breakfasts 60
Tomato Frittata
Roast Beef Cucumber Slices
Sausage Scramble
Ginger-Cranberry Smoothie with
  Smoked Ham and Cheese
Ham-Baked Egg
Italian Omelette
New Orleans Prawn Roll

Which Carbs Lunches 68
Italian Croque Monsieur
Vietnamese Crab Soup
Cajun Prawn Salad
Roast Chicken Vegetable Soup
Rainbow Tomato Plate
Horseradish-Crusted Salmon Salad
Chinese Chicken Salad

Which Carbs Dinners 76
Crispy Cod with Ratatouille
Aubergine Parmesan with Linguine
Mediterranean Steak
Stir-Fried Veal
Five-Spice Tuna Tataki
Chicken with Black Bean Salsa
Veal Piccata

Right Carbs 90
Breakfast
Lunch
Dinner
Right Carbs 14-Day Meal Plan

Right Carbs Breakfasts 94
Ham and Pepper Frittata
Smoked Salmon Sandwich
Strawberry Splash with Cottage
  Cheese-Stuffed Chicory
Microwave Portobello Scramble
Mediterranean Scramble on Toast
Monte Cristo Sandwich
Provençal Omelette

Right Carbs Lunches 102
Mulligatawny Soup
BLT Sandwich on Rye
Layered Antipasto Salad
Blue Cheese and Beef Pasta Salad

Chicory and Orange Salad with
  Swiss Turkey
Mushroom and Sausage Soup
Danish Prawn Smorrebrod

Right Carbs Dinners 110
Roast Pork with Strawberry Salsa
Mahi Mahi Satay with Thai Peanut
  Sauce
Turkey Gratinée with Basil Linguine
Whisky-Soused Salmon
Roasted Pepper and Olive Snapper
Hawaiian Chicken with Pineapple
  Caesar Salad
Mexican Sopes

Super Speed Suppers 124

**Quick Start Super Speed
Suppers 126**
Greek Prawns with Feta Cheese
Jamaican Jerk Pork
Savoury Sage Chicken

**Which Carbs Super Speed
Suppers 130**
Swordfish in Spanish Sofrito Sauce
Peasant Country Soup
Beef Teriyaki with Chinese Noodles

**Right Carbs Super Speed
Suppers 134**
Parmesan Sole
Chicken Creole
Black Bean Soup with Rice
Mock Hungarian Goulash

Weekends 140

**Quick Start Weekend
Meals 142**
Dijon Chicken with Crunchy Couscous
Garlic-Stuffed Steak
Veal Saltimbocca

**Which Carbs Weekend
Meals 148**
Spiced Cowboy Steak
Mediterranean Snapper with
  Provençal Salad
Chicken and Walnuts in Lettuce Puffs
Steak in Port Wine

**Right Carbs Weekend
Meals 156**
Pan-Seared Tuna with Mango Salsa
Indian-Spiced Chicken
Pork Chops with Apple Relish

Entertaining 162

Italian Supper for Friends 164
Garden Crudités
Chicken Tonnato
Lentil and Rice Salad
String Beans with Crumbled
  Gorgonzola
White Chocolate Whip

Dinner Party for Eight 172
Bruschetta
Radicchio, Chicory and Watercress
  Salad
Guinea Fowl in Red Wine
Brown Rice with Toasted Pinenuts
Roasted Asparagus with Red Pepper
Berry Cups with Almond Sauce

Casual Soup Supper 180
Creamy Wild Mushroom Soup
Grilled Halibut Sandwich
Three Bean Salad
Mango Fool

Buffet for Friends 186
Prawns in Lime-Mustard Sauce
Roasted Meat Platter with
  Horseradish and Honey Mustard
  Dressing
Tomato Platter
Pasta Salad
Frozen Yoghurt Berry Cup

Barbecue Party 194
Spicy Tuna Spread
No-Fuss Salad Bar
Lime Barbecued Chicken with Black
  Bean Sauce
Green Bean and Orzo Salad
Melon with Marinated Strawberries

Index 202
Acknowledgments 208

introduction

Seven years ago my husband came home from a visit to the cardiologist and said, 'My doctor wants me to go on a low-carbohydrate diet.' His triglycerides were high and climbing and he was having trouble losing the few pounds he had gained on holiday. This was a new challenge for me. I didn't want to follow the route of gimmick eating: no eating all the eggs and bacon you want or eating at certain times of the day or with certain food combinations. On the other hand, as I watched him struggle to put together low-carb meals, I realised that this was going to be a challenge for both of us. Bagels for breakfast and cans of sugary soft drinks after tennis were out. No more baked potato with his steak. And what could he substitute for crackers and crisps with drinks? I wanted a real eating lifestyle that fitted our busy lives, our eating out, entertaining. Most of all I wanted good food that was good for us, too.

I worked with two cardiologists, an endocrinologist and nutritionists to create an eating lifestyle that was healthy and balanced. What I found was that the doctors and nutritionists could readily explain why this approach worked but could not tell me how to adapt it to my busy life. In fact, when I attended medical lectures with these doctors, the reception for the diet was highly enthusiastic, but the questions at the end – even from the doctors in the audience were – 'How do I do it? What do I eat?' The recipes I created had to be low in carbohydrates, use lean proteins and mono-unsaturated fats (olive and rapeseed oil), and most of all be delicious. The result was my book, *Low-Carb Meals in Minutes*, which was so well received it reached number one on Amazon.com's bestseller list.

What prompted me to write this sequel was the incredible response from readers:

'Your cookbook *Low-Carb Meals in Minutes* was truly an inspiration to me, and I attribute most of my weight loss of 30lb to using your healthy and delicious recipes (husband pleasers as well). Thank you for your wonderful contributions to keeping us well fed in such a healthy manner.'

'Although you have likely heard this a million times, your book is outstanding. I must own close to 50–75 cookbooks I've collected over the years. The way you organised your book with shopping lists and cooking tips, yours is among my favourites.'

'I just want to let you know how well-organised the cookbook is, and how tasty all of the recipes are. I am always very satisfied by the meals. I am still in the Quick Start phase of the book, but have found that the recipes are so varied. I'm surprised that my husband also enjoys them! I see it more as a change in my diet, rather than being "on" a diet. The way your meals are set up forces me to plan things out, and not resort to "quick" fixes. Thanks again for putting together a great cookbook!'

'So many of your menus are part of my daily repertoire now. Tonight we enjoyed "grilled scallops parmigiana" – wonderful! I have tried to plan low-carb meals for three years but with a full-time job as a home economics teacher (which diminishes my desire to cook!) and other obligations, I found that what my husband and I were eating was boring: grilled chicken or fish, vegetables and salad, dinners out or fast food. I know what to do and how to do it but it takes time – you have done all the planning and all I have to do after a day's work is to drop in to the supermarket and I can have a good tasting meal in half an hour or less! What I have enjoyed most are the sauces that accompany the poultry or fish, which deliver great flavour. I have discovered that I must get all the ingredients ready before cooking as the preparation is so quick! My best weeks have been when I have shopped for a whole week and have no decisions about what to make for dinner.'

'My husband and I took part in an office competition to lose weight. We used your book and my husband lost 30lb and I've lost 20. And I've talked to all of my friends about it. We love the recipes. Thanks.'

'Your book is exactly what I've been looking for. My husband is an endocrinologist and has advised his patients about many of the things you discuss.'

'We bought two copies of *Low-Carb Meals in Minutes* and gave one to our daughter and son-in-law. Our particular favourite is the chocolate soufflé dessert. It is hard for me to believe that something so delicious is not bad for you.'

'My husband has high blood pressure and high cholesterol and we are looking for a good diet to follow. This one is the right ticket. Have tried the recipes and love them.'

'So far *Low-Carb Meals in Minutes* has been great for my husband and me, because we used to get tired of eating the same things over and over again, and we never ate healthy foods. Now we are eating much more healthily.'

Low-Carb Meals in Minutes is a three-step programme to losing weight and keeping it off. The first, Quick Start, is a two-week menu that jump-starts quick weight loss. Which Carbs is the next two-week step that gradually reintroduces carbohydrates into the menu while you are still losing weight. The final phase, Right Carbs, is a balanced menu that shows how to eat the right carbohydrates and keep the weight off. *Low-Carb Diet for Life* gives an entirely new two weeks of meals for each of these phases.

A new feature in this book is a Super Speed Supper section containing even quicker dinners for busy week nights, based on buying partially prepared ingredients from the supermarket. The supermarkets have come a long way in helping us get our meals on the table in minutes. For those nights when you want to get dinner ready in 15 minutes, this section has meals based on ingredients bought in the supermarket that can be quickly assembled into a meal at home that fits our guidelines.

Another feature is a Weekends section containing meals that are a little special when you have some additional time. You can enjoy weekend meals and not feel that dreaded Monday morning I-have-to-be-good syndrome.

I have, also, answered the question of how to entertain within the eating lifestyle with five different parties in the Entertaining section. I have created meals that won't break the carb or calorie scale. I had some friends over for dinner and they phoned the next day to say how much they loved the food but were afraid to get on the scales after having seconds. I told them to forget the scales. All of the foods fit the low-carb guidelines, and they didn't have to worry. They couldn't believe it. The Entertaining section here is filled with this style of food. From football parties to a casual dinner with friends to an elegant dinner for eight, you can choose whichever menu suits your needs. And don't tell your guests the food is low-carb or healthy and they'll just enjoy the fun. Finding the time to shop and cook for friends can be difficult these days. The parties in this section use ingredients that can be bought in one-stop shopping at the local supermarket. The recipes take minutes to make and many can be made ahead. I give you a shopping list and countdown explaining how far in advance the recipe can be made, how to store it, and how to reheat and serve it.

While producing my radio programme in Miami, I was surprised that several of the men at the radio station were trying to cut back on their carbohydrates. Their first questions were, 'What's on the list?' and 'What's off the list?'

I myself was lost when I first tried to make low-carbohydrate meals. I had to fundamentally rethink my approach to shopping and cooking. I started by restocking the larder and refrigerator. The changes were dramatic.

Off the list were

- Low-fat processed foods such as fat-free biscuits and cakes and other sugary desserts
- Fat-free mayonnaise, salad dressings, cream cheese and sour cream
- Condiments, sauces and salsas where sugar is one of the first five ingredients
- Pancakes, bagels and waffles
- Jams and jellies
- Pizza and platefuls of pasta as a main course
- Garnished baked potato as a meal
- Sugary soft drinks and fruit juices
- Crisps, pretzels and popcorn

On the list were

- Eggs, as many as four a week (We hadn't eaten them for breakfast in 10 years.)
- Egg substitute (which is basically egg whites), as a good source of protein
- A well-stocked vegetable drawer, including cucumbers, lettuce, celery, sweet peppers, mushrooms and tomatoes
- Lean deli meats, such as turkey breast, chicken, ham and roast beef
- Brown rice and wholemeal pasta, in place of the

lower fibre, less nutritious white varieties

- High-fibre, whole-grain breads that are relatively low in carbs
- No-sugar-added tomato sauce and salad dressings
- Real mayonnaise made with soya bean or olive oil
- High-fibre, no-sugar-added bran cereal for breakfast
- Olive and rapeseed oil
- Walnuts, pecans, almonds and peanuts
- Eight glasses (1.8 litres/3 pints) of water per day

With this list of dos and don'ts, I created recipes that are fast, fun and delicious. My husband's response was enthusiastic: he lost weight, has kept it off for seven years, and lowered his blood cholesterol and triglyceride counts to healthy levels.

Why is this lifestyle becoming mainstream in today's eating? Why are millions of people giving up their sandwiches and pasta meals? After unsuccessful attempts at weight loss from low-fat, high-carb diets, they're finally getting the results they want from a low-carb lifestyle. What are the principles behind it and why is it working for so many people?

In a nutshell, the theory behind low-carbohydrate diets is this: eating lots of carbohydrates over-stimulates insulin production, causing peaks and valleys in blood sugar levels that, in turn, create hunger pangs. On the other hand, protein is digested more slowly, promoting more even blood sugar levels. Eating more protein, fewer carbs, and more mono-unsaturated fat promotes weight loss by decreasing fat storage, increasing fat burning, and delaying the onset of hunger pangs.

The major low-carbohydrate books, such as *The Zone*, *Protein Power*, *Sugar Busters*, *Dr Atkins' New Diet Revolution* and *The Carbohydrate Addict's Diet*, differ in their approaches, but their central idea is to use diet to moderate insulin levels for the reasons explained above. All of the recipes in this book fit into the low-carbohydrate guidelines outlined in these books (and others on the subject).

Several cardiologists steered me away from diets that call for high levels of saturated fat. The menus in this book are similar to a Mediterranean-style diet using fresh vegetables, mono-unsaturated olive and rapeseed oils, and lean meats and fish.

These meals follow the same guidelines as in *Low-Carb Meals in Minutes*: attractive, delicious, fun, healthy, complete meals that are quick and easy to make. All the breakfast, lunch and dinner menus are presented as entire meals, so you don't have to think about how to cook a dish or what goes with what.

I developed these techniques after many years of juggling my family, career (founding and running a cookery school, guiding a gourmet supermarket as its executive director, writing a food column for newspapers and magazines, and hosting a radio talk show), and a desire for good food. It's a method that covers all aspects from purchasing and preparing ingredients to presenting complete meals.

My *Dinner in Minutes* newspaper columns have simple, easy-to-follow recipes. From years of training, I've learned to use classic techniques and familiar combinations to produce delicious results while cutting the cooking time.

It's a blueprint that can be used for everyday meals or dressed up for parties or special occasions.

Special Features

Shopping List

The Low-Carb Diet for Life blueprint contains a shopping list based on how the food is bought in the shops.

- Quick shopping is as important as quick cooking. You won't have to think about how many mushrooms to buy. I've given you the amount.

- list the ingredients by supermarket departments to help you navigate the aisles with ease.

- I've included tips on how to get in and out of the supermarket fast and how to take advantage of today's timesaving prepared foods.

- The shopping list saves you both time and money since you buy only what you need.

- The staples list helps you organise your store cupboards so that they are not filled with extraneous items. To help you plan your stores, I have included a separate section using the staples listed in the book. You will already have many of the ingredients for the recipes and only need to buy a few fresh items.

Shopping Guidelines

Many of the recipes call for prepared condiments such as salad dressings, pasta sauce and Chinese sauces.

- There are many brands to choose from. To help you pick the ones that will fit the nutritional guidelines, I have added a section that tells you what to look for on the nutritional labels of the products.

- Find the products that you like best and keep them on hand so you won't have to think about which one to use.

Helpful Hints and Countdown

Each meal contains helpful hints on shopping, cooking and substitutions, as well as a countdown so you can get the whole meal on the table at the same time.

- You can hit the kitchen on the run without having to plan or think about each step.

- In my home, the dinner preparation encompasses the time I turn on the light in the kitchen until the plates are brought to the table.

- The helpful hints tell you what to buy, how to buy, and what you can substitute. They include tips on the best preparation method and quick-cooking

techniques, as well as timesaving clean-up tips.

- *The Low-Carb Diet for Life* doesn't mean grilled chicken every night. You will find a wide variety of delicious meals covering many ethnic flavours.

- As you eat your way through this book, you can enjoy Tuscan Chicken; Five-Spice Tuna Tataki; Whisky-Soused Salmon; Mahi Mahi Satay with Thai Peanut Sauce; and Mexican Sopes. Wherever I travel throughout the world, I go to street markets with chefs, taste their foods, and bring back their flavours to add to the repertoire of simple, low-carb recipes.

Flexibility

A blueprint means that it is totally flexible.

- When you choose a fish recipe, you can buy the freshest-looking fish in the shop rather than the fish called for in the recipe.

- You can use the best sirloin or fillet steak, or more economical cuts like flank and skirt steaks.

- All of the recipes were tested to produce delicious results with products obtained by one-stop shopping in your local supermarket.

- Branching out to use the freshest and best ingredients, like a favourite gourmet infused olive oil or aged balsamic vinegar, will add even more flavour and zip to these recipes.

- You can use the ingredients called for or change them within the blueprint to suit your taste.
- This flexible approach lets you choose whatever is in season, on sale, or just fits your mood.

As I mentioned above, this low-carbohydrate lifestyle is divided into three phases: an initial phase of significant carbohydrate reduction, an intermediate phase for reintroduction of carbs, and a maintenance phase of balanced eating.

QUICK START – The first step to a successful eating plan calls for a reduction of carbohydrates. While differences exist, most proponents advise a level of about 30–40 grams of carbs a day. My Quick Start section maintains that level through healthy recipes containing vegetables and lean proteins.

WHICH CARBS – Carbohydrates are an important nutrient and the second step reintroduces high-fibre, low-simple-sugar carbohydrates at a level permitting continued weight loss. Listening to the questions from the participants in my low-carb classes, I realised the

returning to higher levels of carbohydrates will negate all of the benefits they've achieved.

RIGHT CARBS – The third stage leaves you permanently with the Right Carbs. So, what should you eat to maintain your weight loss? Right Carbs has the answers. This section achieves a well-balanced lifestyle of approximately 40 per cent calories from carbohydrates, 30 per cent calories from lean proteins, and 30 per cent calories from fat (primarily mono-unsaturated).

So how does my husband handle holidays and blow-out weekends? No need to worry here. Remember, balance is the key. We have found that you can splurge on special occasions without negative effects when you come back to the Right Carbs. In fact, one cardiologist adviser said that varying from a good base once in a while still leaves you much better off than if you don't have that base at all. In other words, the low-carbohydrate approach is forgiving. Following the programme even with some deviations will produce a good result. My husband found that returning to the Right Carbs is easy because it takes so little effort and the menus are so appealing. Any time you want to restart weight loss, you can go back to Quick Start for a week or two and work yourself back up to Right Carbs.

The Low-Carb Diet for Life is for all of you who want to eat healthily and fit a low-carbohydrate weight-loss programme into your time-starved lives. The low-carb lifestyle has certainly changed our lives. My husband and I no longer think about what is and isn't low-carb – we just consider it good food that fits into his busy schedule.

Before you start a programme of this type, it is always best to check with your doctor first. This is especially true if you are taking any medication under a doctor's care. If your doctor recommends a blood test, it will provide a baseline against which to compare your results.

These meals have been made by my many students and readers from all over the United States. Wherever I travel and lecture, they tell me how well they work. I get hundreds of e-mails on how well they're doing and how these easy meals have changed their lives. They love the variety that comes from my travels around the world. My goal in sharing these recipes with you is to help you enjoy good food for good health. My husband and I love good food. Now, with these recipes, we can live to eat and eat to live. We hope you enjoy them too. Bon appétit.

Smart Shopping the Low-Carb Way

'I hate to shop. I'd cook more if I had the ingredients at home,' is a comment I hear often. Here are some tips that will help get you in and out of the shops quickly. It should help you with the I-hate-to-shop syndrome.

Some Advice

The adage of 'Don't go shopping on an empty stomach' is true. It can be a disaster. If I go to the shops when I'm tired and hungry, I just get to a starving point and eat anything offered to me. Go after a meal or have a snack before you go. This will help you concentrate on what you should be buying instead of what you shouldn't buy.

Try to go to the supermarket when it isn't crowded or directly after you've put in a long day's work. Carry a cooler in your car so you can stop on the way to work, during lunch, or at other times. (The cooler will protect foods from moderate heat and cold. It won't help with extreme heat or freezing temperatures.)

Many offices have refrigerators. If one is available to you, shop before work or at lunch and store your food in the refrigerator. Here's a hint: there have been many times when I've left my packages at work or at a friend's house. The best solution to this is to put your car keys in one of the shopping bags. You won't be able to go anywhere without them.

Keep the foods from my staples list on hand. (See page 19.) You will only need to pick up a few fresh items to complete your meal.

Supermarket Savvy

Let the Markets Help You

Supermarkets are constantly updating their product mix to help us get our meals on the table fast. Use the supermarket to your advantage.

Salad Bars

These are great for picking up a quick salad or lunch or buying cut vegetables and fruits for cooking at home.

Deli

Look for new leaner cuts of cooked meats – all with nutritional analysis. Gammon, roast beef and ham have been made leaner and without high carbs.

Dairy

Reduced-fat cheese has come a long way. Gone is the rubbery cheese that won't melt. Many brands using new techniques have developed lower-fat cheeses with flavour and that melt well.

Prepared Foods

Ask for roast chicken breast only. Ask for an ingredients list. Read the labels carefully for all prepared foods. Many have added salt and sugar. Many prepared sauces and condiments are now made in a low-salt, low-carbohydrate version. Look for these in the supermarket. (See page 12 for Shopping Guidelines.)

Fruit and Veg Department

Bags of washed, ready-to-eat salads have been one of the best conveniences I've seen. Read the labels. If they don't say ready-to-eat or washed, then you will need to wash the ingredients prior to using.

Shredded carrots, lettuce and coleslaw mixtures are another big help in getting meals on the table in minutes.

Many supermarkets have cubes of melons and pineapple ready to eat.

Meat Department

Look for lower fat or lean meats. Many stores now have separate sections for lean meats or mark them with special labels.

There are many marinated or pre-cooked meats available. Watch for sugar, salt and fat content.

Roasted chicken breast, strips and pieces are available. The ones without skin or honey sauces are perfect for salads, sandwiches and soups.

Grocery Aisles

There are many items that make our lives easier and more are coming out each day. Low-fat, no-sugar-added tomato sauce, pasta sauces and salad dressings are a few of the products. In fact, there are so many available, it's best to try a few and, when you find one you like, keep a few bottles on hand. Most important is to read the nutritional labels and ingredients lists. (See page 17 for the Shopping Guidelines.)

How to Read the Labels

It's worth a few extra minutes to read the labels on the food you're buying, as many prepared foods have added salt and sugar. However, the terms used can be confusing.

The Food Safety Act of 1990 makes it an offence to falsely describe a food's contents. Other provisions cover specific terms.

'Low-fat' means 3 grams of fat or less per 100g/ml.
'Low-sodium' means 40mg or less per 100g/ml.
'Sugar Free' means 0.2g or less per 100g/ml.
'No added sugar' means no sugar, or foods composed mainly of sugar, is added to the food or its ingredients.
'Light' or 'lite' is not covered by law. This term can be used to describe the texture of a food, or to suggest it is low in fat.

Check the serving size on the label. It can be misleading. If the serving size is 1 tablespoon, you need to think if that is the amount you will actually eat.

Ingredients must be listed in descending order by weight. Generally, if an ingredient is fifth or lower in the list, it has minimal amounts in each serving.

Shopping Guidelines

Throughout the book I use prepared products from the supermarket. There are many brands that will fit the bill but there is considerable variation in their content. The best advice is to find the product that fits the nutritional analysis and has the best flavour. Once you've found one you prefer, keep it on hand.

Here are some guidelines on what to look for on nutritional labels:

Oil and Vinegar Dressing, Balsamic Dressing, Vinaigrettes

The nutritional analysis for meals using one of these ingredients is based on olive oil or rapeseed oil dressings. Try to stay away from non-fat dressings. In general when they cut the fat, they add carbohydrates.

Look for:

Quantity	Calories	Carbohydrates
1 tablespoon	75	0.5–1.5g

Mayonnaise

Look for:

Soya bean oil, rapeseed oil or olive oil (Major brands are made with soya bean oil.)

Quantity	Calories	Carbohydrates
1 tablespoon	100	0g

Reduced Fat Mayonnaise

Look for:

Quantity	Calories	Carbohydrates	Fat
1 tablespoon	50	1g	5g

Caesar Dressing

Look for:

Quantity	Calories	Carbohydrates
1 tablespoon	80	0.5–1.5g

Tomato and Pasta Sauces

Look for no-sugar-added, no-salt-added, or low-sodium brands. There are many excellent ones to choose from.

Look for:

Quantity	Calories	Carbohydrates	Fibre	Sodium	Fat
225ml (8fl oz)	60–80	12–14g	2–3g	40mg	0g

Non-fat, Low-Sodium Chicken Stock

Look for:

Quantity	Calories	Sodium
225ml (8 fl oz)	15	560mg

Low-Sodium Soy Sauce

Look for:

Quantity	Calories	Sodium
1 tablespoon	10	574mg

Tortilla

Look for:

Quantity	Calories	Carbohydrates
15cm (6in) tortilla weighing 25g (1oz)	90	16g

Wholemeal Bread

Look for:

Quantity	Calories	Carbohydrates	Fibre
1 slice	50	10g	3g

Other Breads and Rolls

Look for:

Quantity	Calories	Carbohydrates	Fibre
1 slice/1 roll	80	15g	0.7–2g

Bran Cereal*

Look for:

Quantity	Calories	Carbohydrates	Fibre
25g (1oz)	80	24g	13g

*Read labels carefully; labels say cereals are healthy, but look for the amounts of sugar, syrup or honey.

Lean Ham and Gammon

Look for:

Quantity	Calories	Sodium	Fat
25g (1oz)	37	246mg	1.4g

Reduced-Fat, Semi-Skimmed Milk Mozzarella Cheese

Look for:

Quantity	Calories	Fat	Sodium
25g (1oz)	72	4.5g	132mg

Peppers

Look for:

Quantity	Calories	Carbohydrates	Fat	Sodium
225g (8oz)	40	8g	0g	20mg

Marinated Artichoke Hearts

Look for:

Quantity	Calories	Carbohydrates	Fat	Sodium
25g (1oz)	25	2g	1.5g	90mg

Unsweetened Apple Sauce

Look for:

Quantity	Calories	Carbohydrates	Sodium
225ml (8fl oz)	100	30g	30mg

Low-Fat Frozen Yoghurt

Look for:

Quantity	Calories	Fat	Carbohydrates
115ml (4fl oz)	120	3g	20g

Staples

This is a comprehensive list of the staples listed in the recipes. Keep these staples on hand and you'll only need to pick up a few fresh items to make quick meals.

Tinned or Bottled Goods

Dijon mustard

Fat-free, low-salt chicken stock

Low-sodium tomato or V-8 juice

Low-sodium, no-sugar-added tomato sauce and diced tomatoes

Mayonnaise made with olive or soya bean oil

No-sugar-added olive oil and vinegar dressing

No-sugar-added tomato salsa

Reduced-fat mayonnaise

Tinned chickpeas, black beans, haricot beans, cannellini beans

Tinned tuna packed in water

Condiments

Hot pepper sauce

Low-sodium soy sauce

Worcestershire sauce

Dairy

Butter

Egg substitute

Eggs

Non-fat yoghurt

Parmesan cheese

Skimmed milk

Dry Goods

Artificial sweetener

Cornflour

High-fibre, no-sugar-added bran cereal

Oatmeal

Salt

Wholemeal flour

Wholemeal pasta

Freezer Goods

Frozen chopped onion

Frozen diced green pepper

Grains and Breads

Brown rice (30-minute quick-cooking and 10-minute quick-cooking)

100% wholemeal bread

Lentils

Multi-grain bread

Rye bread

Wholemeal pitta bread

Wholemeal tortilla

Wild rice

Oils and Vinegars

Balsamic vinegar

Distilled white vinegar

Olive oil

Olive oil spray

Rapeseed oil

Red wine vinegar

Rice vinegar

Fruit and Veg Department

Carrots

Celery

Garlic

Lemon

Red onions

Yellow onions

Spices and Herbs

Black peppercorns

Cayenne pepper

Chilli powder

Dried chopped sage

Dried dill

Dried oregano

Dried rosemary

Dried tarragon

Dried thyme

Freeze-dried chives

Grated nutmeg

Ground cinnamon

Ground cumin

Equipment

You really don't need a lot of special equipment to make these meals. However, here's a list of some items that will speed your preparation and cooking and make your life easier.

Food Processor

A food processor or mini-chopper will help quickly slice and chop and also blend foods together.

Garlic Press

Some of the newer ones allow you to crush garlic without peeling the cloves. I also use it to crush fresh ginger.

Knives

Sharp knives are important for fast and accurate cutting. A blunt knife can be dangerous. It can slip or slide when you are trying to slice. Three different types are all you really need for most cutting tasks: a 10cm (4in) paring knife, a 20cm (8in) chef's knife and a small serrated knife for fruit or tomatoes.

Meat Thermometer

I love the new style that uses a probe. The cord is connected to a dial that sits on the work surface. The dial is easy to read and doesn't get hot or dirty. With the cord, it works well for items on the stove, in the oven, or under the grill.

Microwave Ovens

Use this fast-cooking appliance. And remember, any dish that's microwave safe is dishwasher safe, too. Be careful; it's easy to overcook food. Food continues to cook several seconds after it has been removed from the oven.

Pots and Pans

You can make most of the meals in this book using a medium 23–25cm (9–10in) non-stick frying pan, a large 3–4 litre (5–7 pint) saucepan and a wok. Non-stick frying pans are essential, as these recipes are designed using small amounts of oil. If you follow the instructions, your food will not stick.

Scales

Small kitchen scales are very handy and not expensive.

Vegetable Peeler

For easy peeling, make sure yours is sharp. These are actually little knives and should be replaced as they start to get blunt.

Quick Cooking Tips and Helpful Hints

Each recipe has a Helpful Hints section. Knowing what to substitute, the best way to prepare ingredients, or some other shortcut can make a big difference to the time it takes to get your meal on the table.

Chopping Fresh Herbs

To quickly chop herbs, snip the leaves off the stem with scissors.

Crisp Stir-Fry

For crisp, not steamed, stir-fried vegetables, make sure your wok or frying pan is very hot. The oil should be smoking. Let the vegetables sit a minute before tossing to allow the wok to regain its heat.

Dried Spices and Herbs

If using dried spices, make sure the jar is less than 6 months old. To bring out the flavour of the dried herbs, chop them with fresh parsley. The juice from the parsley will help release the flavour of the herbs.

Electric Cooking

To get a quick high/low response from electric rings, heat two rings, one on medium-high and the other on low. Move the pan back and forth between them.

Fluffy Rice

I like to cook my rice like pasta, using a saucepan of boiling water that's large enough for the rice to roll freely. Use this method or follow the directions on the rice packet.

Food Processor

To use the food processor for a recipe without having to stop to wash the bowl, first chop the dry ingredients (such as nuts), and then the wet ones (such as onion). You won't have to stop in the middle of preparing the ingredients.

Fresh Ginger

To chop fresh ginger quickly, cut it into small cubes and press through a garlic press with large holes. If using a press with small holes, just capture the juice that is squeezed out; it will give enough flavour for the recipe.

Parmesan Cheese

Buy good-quality Parmesan cheese and grate it yourself or chop it in the food processor. Freeze extra for quick use later. You can quickly spoon out what you need and leave the rest frozen.

Peeling Prawns

Buying peeled prawns saves time otherwise spent shelling them yourself.

Slices and Weight

To determine the weight of sliced cheese or packaged meats, look at the packet weight or nutritional analysis to determine how much each slice weighs.

Timely Stir-Fry

To keep from looking back at a recipe as you stir-fry the ingredients, line them up on a chopping board or plate in the order of use. You will know which ingredient comes next.

Washing Herbs

The quickest way to wash watercress, rocket, parsley or basil is to place the bunch, head first, into a bowl of water. Leave for a minute, then lift out and shake dry. The dirt and sand will be left behind.

Washing Mushrooms

To clean whole mushrooms, wipe them with damp kitchen paper.

Tips for Eating Out

One of the biggest challenges to making sure we eat healthily is that 60 per cent of our meals are prepared outside the home. We eat out, bring in and eat on the run. Use the recipes in this book as a guide to eating out. Once you understand the types of food and proportion sizes, you will be able to order from the menu with confidence. Here are some hints and tips to eat well in spite of your schedule:

● Avoid all deep-fried foods.

● Avoid sugary drinks. Opt for water, unsweetened iced tea or diet drinks.

● Plain, soft tacos or tortilla-filled wraps are fine as long as they aren't filled with rice and beans. Ask for wholemeal, if possible.

● Roasted or grilled meats are best. Make sure you include vegetables with your meal. Stay away from sugar-based sauces, especially barbecue sauce and most glazes.

● Many meals are loaded with carbs. Order two vegetables instead of a starch. Most restaurants are used to substituting this way.

● Ask for your salad dressing on the side. Most salads come swimming in dressing. You'll be surprised how far 1 tablespoon of dressing will go. Or just dip your vegetables into the dressing on the side.

● If you order dessert, share it with the table or make sure you don't have a starch during dinner. Better still, order a fresh fruit salad or berries.

● Have a low-carb snack (vegetables, a few nuts, a slice of low-carbohydrate cheese) before you go out to eat. This will help you avoid the basket of bread on the table while you're waiting for your meal.

● Ask for the bread basket to be brought to the table with the main course to save munching on the bread while you are ordering.

● Don't go out for drinks on an empty stomach. One drink will make you hungry, and you'll eat the first thing you can find. Have a healthy snack before you go out. (See page 25 for a snack list.) If you think it will be a long night, start with sparkling water with a piece of lemon or lime or a diet soft drink first.

- Fast food can be fine. Order grilled chicken or fish and discard the bread. Or eat it as an open sandwich using half a roll. Order a salad with the dressing on the side. Stay away from chips, baked potatoes and crisps.

- Chinese food can be loaded with sugar. Order stir-fried meats and vegetables or skewered meats, and avoid soups with wontons. Avoid egg rolls, ribs in thick sauce and noodles. It is refreshing to see that some restaurants are offering brown rice as an alternative to white rice.

- Italian food doesn't have to mean a plate of pasta. Order an antipasto platter or any of the meats, salads or vegetables.

- French food can be very healthy. Order clear soups, salads, vegetables, meats or seafood, but avoid heavy sauces and bread.

- Japanese sushi is based on rice – very often with sugar added to it. Try miso soup or any of the cooked meats and vegetables instead.

- Mexican food can be high in saturated fat and carbohydrates. Fajitas (1 tortilla) with the garnishes, grilled meats and salads are fine. Avoid rice, refried beans and nachos.

SIZING IT UP

Watch portion size when eating out. Many restaurant servings are large enough for two meals. Here's a guide to help you size up what you should be eating.

75g (3oz) cooked meat, poultry, or fish	a deck of cards
40g (1oz) cheese	6 dice
1 tortilla	a 18-cm (7-inch) plate
1 muffin	a large egg
1 teaspoon butter	a thumb tip
2 tablespoons peanut butter	a golf ball

Information from *Food Insight News* published by IFIC (International Food Information Council)

Quick Snacks

Snacks are important little meals that will help you through the day, especially during the first Quick Start phase. They can prevent that sinking feeling at 4 or 5 p.m. when your energy is low, or the mid-morning, is-it-time-for-lunch clock watching.

Knowing what to snack on and how to have it handy can help prevent raids on the vending machine to satiate sweet cravings.

Here are some ideas:

The remains of an extra large lunch salad, which you can take back to your office or home

- 25g (1oz) low-fat cheese (mozzarella, small round individually packed wax-covered low-fat cheese)

- 50ml (2fl oz) low-fat cottage cheese

- 25g (1oz) nuts, such as almonds, pecans and walnuts. Keep small packets of nuts, the type that are found in the baking section of the supermarket, in your drawer at work, handbag or briefcase. They're easy to carry around and contain portion-size amounts.

- 50g (2oz) deli meats, such as lean ham, turkey, chicken or roast beef

- 1 hard-boiled egg. Keep a few hard-boiled eggs on hand for snacks. They will need to be refrigerated at the office.

- 25g (1oz) sunflower seeds

- 6 olives

- Any vegetables such as cucumber slices, celery sticks, broccoli or cauliflower florets and sliced pepper

quick start

THIS TWO-WEEK MEAL PLAN IS DESIGNED TO START YOU OFF ON CUTTING CARBS FROM YOUR MEALS.

When I give cooking classes and show these meals, the response always surprises me. 'You mean I can eat all of that?' is the usual response. Knowing the quantities of each type of food you can eat will help you to build your own recipes to fit your lifestyle.

I have organised the menus into a meal-at-a-glance chart with some easy and quick meals mid-week and those that take a little more time for the weekends. They are arranged to give variety throughout the day and over the days of the week.

Breakfast

There's plenty of variety in these breakfasts to fit all tastes, from Microwave Marinara Scramble to Turkey Salsa Roll. Pick the ones you like and use them for this two-week period.

Mid-Morning Snack

When you first start reducing carbs, you will need to eat a mid-morning snack. I've included a section with some suggestions. (See page 25.)

Lunch

There's a lunch for any occasion here – quick-take lunches that can be eaten at home or taken with you, more elaborate lunches for when you have more time or friends come round.

Enjoy Spanish Tuna-Stuffed Tomatoes and Nutty Chicken Minestrone. These meals can be made at home and taken to work. They are commonly found on most lunch menus. If you are eating out, use these recipes as a guide for the portions you should eat.

I usually order my salads with the dressing on the side. Most salads come swimming in dressing. I find that 1 tablespoon of dressing gently coats the salad without overpowering it. So, I prefer to add the dressing to the salad myself. (See pages 23–24 for more tips on eating out.)

Mid-Afternoon Snack

When you first start reducing carbs, you will need to eat a mid-afternoon snack. (See page 25.)

Dinner

Do you feel like Italian, French or American food tonight? There's something from each ethnic group – Tuscan Chicken, Roasted Salmon and Herb Sauce, and Chicken Burgers with Warm Mushroom Salad are some of the tempting meals.

For those days when you are really pressed for time, select Savoury Sage Chicken or Jamaican Jerk Pork from the Super Speed Suppers section of the book.

For weekends when you have more time and want something special try, the Dijon Chicken with Crunchy Couscous or Garlic-Stuffed Steak from the Weekends section of the book.

How low is low carb? It's important to reduce carbohydrate intake low enough for a period of time so that you eliminate the peaks of insulin secretion. Following the Quick Start 14-Day Meal Plan, you will consume an average of 35–45 grams of carbohydrates per day. Carbohydrate percentage is based on carbohydrates less fibre consumed, which is the normal way of calculating carbohydrate consumption. The balance of these meals is 11 per cent of calories from carbs, 40 per cent of calories from low-fat proteins, and 36 per cent of calories from mono-unsaturated fat and 11 per cent of calories from saturated fat.

To achieve the correct balance, I have structured the recipes as complete meals. Whatever meal you pick, it's best to stay with the entire menu given.

quick start 14-day plan at a glance

week 1	breakfast	lunch	dinner
sunday	Bacon and Cheese Crêpes 31	Sicilian Baked Mushrooms and Sausage 39	Dijon Chicken with Crunchy Couscous 143
monday	Microwave Eggs Parmesan....................32	Chicken with Dill Mustard......................40	Greek Prawns with Feta Cheese 127
tuesday	Mushroom, Turkey and Tarragon Omelette........33	Cheese and Chicken Bundles......................41	Hot Pepper Prawns.......47
wednesday	Turkey Salsa Roll...........34	Nutty Chicken Minestrone 42	Mediterranean Baked Fish............................48
thursday	Microwave Marinara Scramble.....................35	Spanish Tuna-Stuffed Tomatoes......................43	Savoury Sage Chicken......................129
friday	Smoked Salmon -Stuffed Celery..........................36	Crunchy Oriental Chicken Salad............................44	Jamaican Jerk Pork........128
saturday	Sausage and Artichoke Frittata..........................37	Crab Gratin....................45	Chicken Burgers with Warm Mushroom Salad..........50

week 2	breakfast	lunch	dinner
sunday	Bacon and Cheese Crêpes 31	Sicilian Baked Mushrooms and Sausage.................39	Garlic Stuffed-Steak 144
monday	Microwave Eggs Parmesan.....................32	Chicken with Dill Mustard.......................40	Crab Cakes and Slaw......................51
tuesday	Mushroom, Turkey and Tarragon Omelette........33	Cheese and Chicken Bundles.......................41	Pork Escalopes with Spinach and Mushrooms..................52
wednesday	Turkey Salsa Roll...........34	Nutty Chicken Minestrone...................42	Roasted Salmon and Herb Sauce..........................53
thursday	Microwave Marinara Scramble......................35	Spanish Tuna-Stuffed Tomatoes......................43	Tuscan Chicken............54
friday	Smoked Salmon-Stuffed Celery...........................36	Crunchy Oriental Chicken Salad............................44	Savoury Sage Chicken.......................129
saturday	Sausage and Artichoke Frittata.........................37	Crab Gratin...................45	Veal Saltimbocca...........146

quick start
breakfasts

bacon and cheese crêpes

Making eggs into thin crêpes is the secret to this dish. Be sure to use a good non-stick frying pan for best results.

bacon and cheese crêpes

225ml (8fl oz) egg substitute

Freshly ground black pepper

Olive oil spray

175g (6oz) lean gammon, cut into 2.5cm (1in) strips

75g (3oz) grated semi-skimmed milk mozzarella cheese

1 medium tomato, sliced

Pre-heat grill. Mix egg substitute with pepper to taste. Heat a medium non-stick frying pan on medium-high heat. Spray with olive oil spray and pour half the egg substitute into frying pan and spread to make a thin layer. Leave to cook for 2 minutes. Turn over for 1 minute. Remove from heat to a foil-lined baking tray. Repeat with second half of egg mixture. Sprinkle bacon and cheese over crêpes. Fold over once and place under grill about 25cm (10in) from heat. Grill for 2 minutes or until cheese melts. Carefully slide on to a plate, place sliced tomatoes on the side and serve.

Makes 2 servings.

Per serving: 335 calories, 43.2 grams protein, 7.0 grams carbohydrate, 14.2 grams fat (7.5 saturated), 73 milligrams cholesterol, 1227 milligrams sodium, 0 grams fibre

helpful hint

- Make these crêpes ahead, and fill and warm in a microwave oven when needed.

countdown

- Pre-heat grill.
- Make egg base.
- Complete recipe.

shopping list

FRUIT AND VEG

1 medium tomato

DAIRY

1 packet grated semi-skimmed milk mozzarella cheese

DELI

175g (6oz) lean gammon

STAPLES

Egg substitute

Olive oil spray

Black peppercorns

helpful hints

● Buy good-quality Parmesan cheese and grate it yourself or chop it in the food processor. Freeze extra for quick use. You can quickly spoon out what you need and leave the rest frozen.

countdown

● Make eggs.
● Arrange salad on 2 plates.

shopping list

FRUIT AND VEG
1 medium tomato
1 small head romaine lettuce
DELI
110g (4oz) smoked turkey
STAPLES
Eggs (6 needed)
Parmesan cheese
Salt
Black peppercorns

microwave eggs parmesan

Here is another quick microwave breakfast. The timing of this dish depends on the power of your microwave oven. Also, some like their eggs dry, others wet. Select the timing according to your preference. Remember the eggs will continue to cook for about 1 minute after they are removed from the oven.

microwave eggs parmesan

4 egg whites
2 large eggs
110g (4oz) smoked turkey, cut into small cubes
2 tablespoons grated Parmesan cheese
Salt and freshly ground black pepper
Several romaine lettuce leaves
1 medium tomato, sliced

Place 2 egg whites and 1 whole egg in a microwave-safe bowl about 18cm (7in) in diameter. Add 2 tablespoons turkey, 1 tablespoon Parmesan cheese and salt and pepper to taste. Whisk with a fork. Microwave on high for 1 minute. Stir and microwave for 30 seconds and stir. For drier eggs, microwave 30 seconds more. Arrange lettuce leaves on 2 plates and place tomato slices on top. Spoon eggs on to plate. Using the same bowl, repeat for second serving.
Makes 2 servings.

Per serving: 255 calories, 35.3 grams protein, 4.5 grams carbohydrate, 10.9 grams fat (4.0 saturated), 260 milligrams cholesterol, 394 milligrams sodium, 0.2 grams fibre

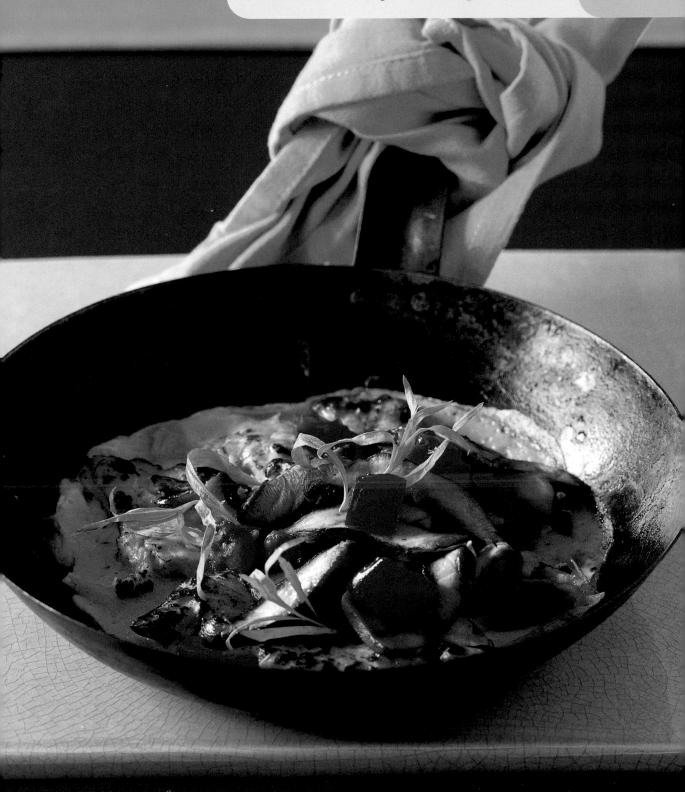

Mushroom, Turkey and Tarragon Omelette   **p33**

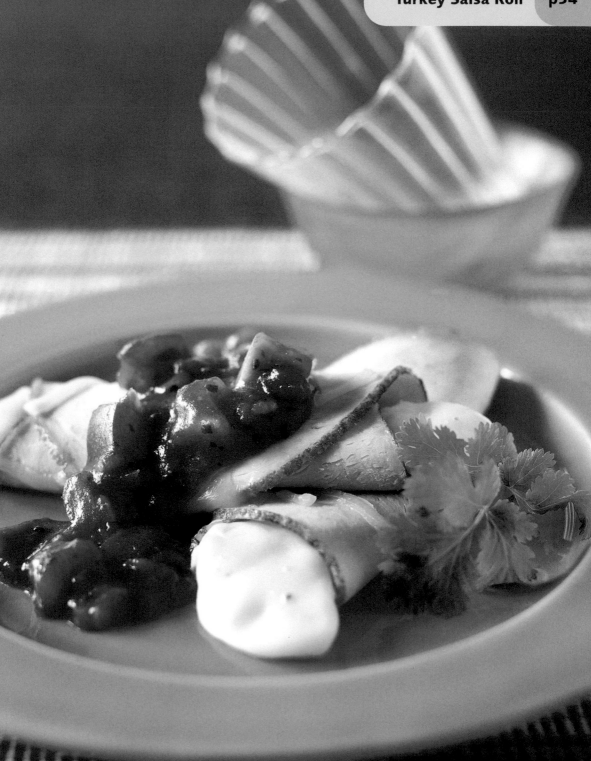

Turkey Salsa Roll   **p34**

mushroom, turkey and tarragon omelette

Omelettes take only minutes to make. A perfect omelette is golden on the top with a delicate creamy centre. The secret is to cook it over medium-high heat for only a couple of minutes.

mushroom, turkey and tarragon omelette

4 egg whites

2 large whole eggs

110g (4oz) smoked turkey breast,
    cut into 25cm (1in) cubes

1 teaspoon dried tarragon

Salt and freshly ground black
    pepper

Olive oil spray

110g (4oz) thinly sliced portobello
    mushrooms

1 medium tomato, cut into 25cm
    (1in) pieces

Place eggs and egg whites in a bowl and stir in turkey, tarragon and salt and pepper to taste. Heat a medium non-stick frying pan over medium-high heat and spray with olive oil. Sauté mushrooms and tomatoes for 2 minutes and remove. Pour in the egg mixture. Let the eggs set for about 30 seconds. Tip the pan and lightly move the eggs so that they set completely. Cook for 1½ minutes or until eggs are set. Cook a few seconds longer for firmer eggs.

Place the mushrooms and tomatoes on half the omelette and fold the omelette in half. Slide out of the pan by tipping the pan and holding a plate vertically against the side of the pan. Turn pan and plate to invert the omelette on to the plate. Cut in half and serve on 2 plates.
Makes 2 servings.

Per serving: 228 calories, 31.5 grams protein,
4.7 grams carbohydrate, 9.3 grams fat (2.5 saturated),
253 milligrams cholesterol, 215 milligrams sodium,
0 grams fibre

helpful hints

- *Any herb can be used.*
- *Dried tarragon is called for in the recipe. If using dried herbs, make sure the jar is less than 6 months old.*
- *For best results, use a good-quality non-stick pan.*

countdown

- *Prepare ingredients.*
- *Complete omelette.*

shopping list

FRUIT AND VEG
    110g (4oz) portobello
    mushrooms
    1 medium tomato
DELI
    110g (4oz) smoked turkey
    breast
STAPLES:
    Eggs (6 needed)
    Olive oil spray
    Dried tarragon
    Salt
    Black peppercorns

turkey salsa roll

Sliced turkey roll stuffed with Cheddar cheese and topped with salsa is a breakfast that can be made ahead and warmed in 1 minute in a microwave oven before eating.

turkey salsa roll

225g (8oz) sliced, smoked turkey breast
50g (2oz) grated reduced-fat Cheddar cheese
225ml (8fl oz) no-sugar-added tomato salsa

Place turkey slices on the work surface or a plate and sprinkle each slice with cheese. Roll up slices and divide between 2 plates. Microwave each plate on high for 1 minute or until cheese melts. If not using a microwave oven, place turkey rolls on a foil-lined baking sheet under a grill for 1 minute. Remove plates from microwave and spoon salsa over the top.
Makes 2 servings.

Per serving: 310 calories, 44.0 grams protein, 10.4 grams carbohydrate, 8.5 grams fat (4.2 saturated), 90 milligrams cholesterol, 1036 milligrams sodium, 4.0 grams fibre

helpful hints

- To help the morning rush, stuff the turkey the night before and warm just before eating.

countdown

- Prepare ingredients.
- Complete dish.

shopping list

DAIRY
1 small packet grated reduced-fat Cheddar cheese
STAPLES:
1 small jar no-sugar-added tomato salsa

microwave marinara scramble

This breakfast takes just minutes to make in a microwave oven. A rich, thick marinara sauce gives these scrambled eggs a taste of Naples.

The timing of this dish depends on the power of your microwave oven. Also, some like their eggs dry, others wet. Select the timing according to your preference. Remember the eggs will continue to cook for about 1 minute after they are removed from the oven.

microwave marinara scramble

150g (5oz) washed, ready-to-eat
   baby spinach
110g (4oz) lean ham, cut into
   2.5cm (1in) pieces
225ml (8fl oz) egg substitute
50ml (2fl oz) low-salt, no-sugar-
   added marinara sauce
Salt and freshly ground black
   pepper
6 tablespoons grated semi-
   skimmed milk mozzarella
   cheese

Place spinach and ham in a microwave-safe bowl and microwave on high for 2 minutes. Divide between 2 plates.

Combine egg substitute and marinara sauce together in a microwave-safe bowl. Season with salt and pepper to taste. Cover with clingfilm or a plate. Microwave on high for 4 minutes. Stir and divide in half. Place each portion on top of the spinach and ham. Sprinkle 2 tablespoons mozzarella cheese on top of each portion. *Makes 2 servings.*

Per serving: 250 calories, 33.6 grams protein, 10.6 grams carbohydrate, 8.6 grams fat (4.0 saturated), 43 milligrams cholesterol, 1127 milligrams sodium, 3.6 grams fibre

helpful hints

● *If you don't have a microwave oven, sauté the spinach for 1 minute in a small frying pan and remove to a plate. Scramble the eggs in the same pan.*

● *If baby spinach is unavailable, use any type of spinach or lettuce.*

countdown

● *Microwave spinach.*
● *Microwave scrambled eggs.*

shopping list

FRUIT AND VEG
   1 bag washed, ready-to-eat baby spinach (150g/5oz needed)
DAIRY
   1 small packet grated semi-skimmed milk mozzarella cheese
DELI
   110g (4oz) lean ham
GROCERY
   1 small jar low-salt, no-sugar-added marinara sauce

staples

   Egg substitute (225ml/8fl oz needed)
   Salt
   Black peppercorns

smoked salmon-stuffed celery

If you're in a hurry, make this breakfast the night before and take it with you to eat on the run.

helpful hints

- *A quick way to cut chives is to snip them with scissors.*
- *Freeze-dried chives can be used instead of fresh.*

countdown

- *Prepare ingredients.*
- *Assemble dish.*

shopping list

FRUIT AND VEG

1 small bunch chives

DAIRY

1 small pot soured cream

SEAFOOD

350g (12oz) smoked salmon

STAPLES:

Celery

Black peppercorns

smoked salmon-stuffed celery

350g (12oz) smoked salmon
50ml (2fl oz) soured cream
2 tablespoons snipped chives
Freshly ground black pepper
8 medium celery stalks

Chop salmon. This can be done in a food processor or by hand. Mix with the soured cream and chives. Add black pepper to taste. Spread into celery and cut stalks into 5cm (2in) pieces. Divide between 2 plates.
Makes 2 servings.

> Per serving: 290 calories, 33.4 grams protein, 13.2 grams carbohydrate, 13.9 grams fat (4.9 saturated), 53 milligrams cholesterol, 1625 milligrams sodium, 4.0 grams fibre

sausage and artichoke frittata

Plump, juicy frittatas take about 15 minutes to make. They can be made ahead and eaten at room temperature or reheated in a microwave oven. They differ from omelettes. An omelette is cooked fast over high heat making it creamy and runny, while a frittata is cooked slowly over low heat, making it firm and set. A frittata needs to be cooked on both sides. Some people flip it in the pan. A much easier way is to place it in a pre-heated oven to finish cooking or under the grill for half a minute.

   Low-fat turkey sausages are available in the supermarkets. If you have a local butcher who makes his own sausages you may be able to pick different flavourings, ranging from mild to spicy hot. Choose whichever type suits your palate.

sausage and artichoke frittata

2 teaspoons olive oil
2 low-fat turkey sausages, cut into 1cm (1/2in) slices (175g/6oz)
4 egg whites
2 large whole eggs
150g (5oz) drained marinated artichoke hearts, cut in half
1 tablespoon freeze-dried chives
Salt and freshly ground black pepper

Pre-heat oven to 200ºC/400ºF/gas mark 6. Heat olive oil in an 18–20cm (7–8in) non-stick frying pan on medium-high heat. Sauté sausage for 3 minutes. Mix egg whites, whole eggs and artichokes together. Add chives and salt and pepper to taste. Reduce heat to medium and pour egg mixture into pan. Spread to cover sausage and artichokes. Leave to set on the bottom for 3 minutes. Place in oven for 7 minutes or until eggs set. If you like drier eggs, leave for 1 further minute.
Makes 2 servings.

Per serving: 337 calories, 29.0 grams protein, 7.0 grams carbohydrate, 21.3 grams fat (4.2 saturated), 258 milligrams cholesterol, 893 milligrams sodium, 1.0 grams fibre

helpful hints

● Egg substitute can be used instead of 2 whole eggs and 6 egg whites.

countdown

● Pre-heat oven to 200ºC/400ºF/gas mark 6.
● Prepare ingredients.
● Make frittata.

shopping list

MEAT
   1 small packet low-fat turkey sausages (175g/6oz needed)
GROCERY
   1 small jar marinated artichoke hearts
   1 small container freeze-dried chives
STAPLES:
   Eggs (6 needed)
   Olive oil
   Salt
   Black peppercorns

quick start
lunches

sicilian baked mushrooms and sausage

Mushrooms baked with garlic and sausage and topped with cheese and breadcrumbs is a dish that originates from Palermo in Sicily. The dish can be baked in an oven or takes only minutes in a microwave.

sicilian baked mushrooms and sausage

Olive oil spray

350g (12oz) low-fat turkey sausages, cut into 2.5cm (1in) pieces

275g (10oz) thinly sliced button mushrooms

4 garlic cloves, crushed

⅛ teaspoon crushed chillies

Salt and freshly ground black pepper

15g (½oz) chopped fresh parsley

2 tablespoons breadcrumbs

3 tablespoons grated Parmesan cheese

Spray a 25cm (10in) microwave-safe pie plate with olive oil spray. Add the sausages and microwave on high for 2 minutes. Remove from microwave and pour off fat. Add mushrooms, garlic and chilli. Add salt and pepper to taste. Sprinkle parsley over mushrooms. Sprinkle breadcrumbs and Parmesan cheese on top. Microwave on high for 5 minutes. Or place in a pre-heated 200ºC/400ºF/gas mark 6 oven for 15 minutes. Divide between 2 plates.
Makes 2 servings.

Per serving: 388 calories, 33.7 grams protein, 11.2 grams carbohydrate, 21.5 grams fat (7.0 saturated), 94 milligrams cholesterol, 1273 milligrams sodium, 0 grams fibre

helpful hints

- *Any combination of mushrooms can be used.*
- *Buy sliced mushrooms or slice in a food processor.*
- *Crushed chillies can be found in the spice section of the supermarket.*
- *Buy good-quality Parmesan cheese and grate it yourself or chop it in the food processor. Freeze extra for quick use. You can spoon out what you need and leave the rest frozen.*

countdown

- *If using an oven, pre-heat to 200ºC/400ºF/gas mark 6.*
- *Prepare ingredients.*
- *Make mushrooms.*

shopping list

FRUIT AND VEG

275g (10oz) button mushrooms, sliced

1 small bunch fresh parsley

MEAT

350g (12oz) low-fat turkey sausages

GROCERY

1 small jar crushed chillies

1 small container plain breadcrumbs

STAPLES:

Olive oil spray

Parmesan cheese

Garlic

Salt

Black peppercorns

chicken with dill mustard

This lunch of sliced chicken breast topped with a dill mustard sauce and crunchy sliced celery requires no cooking and can be assembled the night before. It's also a good recipe for leftover chicken.

chicken with dill mustard

350g (12oz) thick-sliced (about
    0.5cm/¼in) deli chicken breast
3 tablespoons Dijon mustard
1½ tablespoons mayonnaise
1½ teaspoons dried dill
12 medium celery stalks, thinly
    sliced

Divide chicken between 2 plates. Mix mustard, mayonnaise and dill together and spread half the mixture over the chicken. Place celery slices on top and cover with remaining sauce.
Makes 2 servings.

Per serving: 440 calories, 57.9 grams protein,
19.4 grams carbohydrate, 18.5 grams fat
(2.9 saturated), 148 milligrams cholesterol,
1146 milligrams sodium, 6.0 grams fibre

helpful hints

● Dried dill is called for in the recipe. If using dried herbs, make sure the jar is less than 6 months old.

countdown

● Prepare ingredients.
● Complete dish.

shopping list

DELI
    350g (12oz) thick-sliced
        (about 0.5cm/¼in) deli
        chicken breast
STAPLES
    Celery (12 stalks needed)
    Dijon mustard
    Dried dill
    Mayonnaise

cheese and chicken bundles

Roasted chicken, blue cheese, walnuts and yoghurt blend together to make a tasty spread that is rolled into lettuce leaves. These little bundles can be made ahead and taken to eat on the run.

cheese and chicken bundles

50g (2oz) blue cheese, crumbled
50ml (2fl oz) non-fat natural
    yoghurt
2 tablespoons walnut pieces
225g (8oz) roasted chicken strips
Several romaine lettuce leaves
    (about 6)
4 medium celery stalks

Place blue cheese, yoghurt, walnuts and chicken in the bowl of a food processor fitted with a chopping blade. Process to a spreadable consistency. Place lettuce leaves on work surface or a board and spread chicken mixture on leaves. Roll up lengthways and wrap in foil or greaseproof paper. Cut celery stalks into 5cm (2in) pieces and serve on the side.
Makes 2 servings.

Per serving: 411 calories, 46.9 grams protein, 13.3 grams carbohydrate, 21.3 grams fat (7.2 saturated), 118 milligrams cholesterol, 652 milligrams sodium, 3.2 grams fibre

helpful hints

- *Any large lettuce leaves can be used.*
- *Buy plain roasted chicken strips. Stay away from honey roasted or barbecue chicken.*

countdown

- *Prepare ingredients.*
- *Make bundles.*

shopping list

FRUIT AND VEG
    1 small head romaine lettuce
DAIRY
    1 small pot non-fat natural yoghurt
    1 small packet blue cheese
MEAT
    1 packet roasted chicken strips (225g/8oz needed)
GROCERY
    1 small packet walnut pieces
STAPLES
    Celery

nutty chicken minestrone

helpful hints

- Walnuts, pecans or almonds can be substituted for pistachio nuts.
- Buy good-quality Parmesan cheese and grate it yourself or chop it in the food processor. Freeze extra for quick use. You can spoon out what you need and leave the rest frozen.
- Grated carrots are available in the fruit and veg section of the supermarket.

countdown

- Prepare ingredients.
- Make soup.

shopping list

FRUIT AND VEG
  1 small pack grated carrots
  1 bag washed, ready-to-eat spinach
  1 medium tomato
  1 small bunch basil
MEAT
  225g (8oz) roasted chicken strips or pieces
GROCERY
  1 small packet shelled pistachio nuts
STAPLES
  Olive oil
  Parmesan cheese
  Fat-free, low-sodium chicken stock (350ml/12fl oz needed)
  Celery
  Salt
  Black peppercorns

This minestrone is a refreshing blend of flavours using fresh vegetables, chicken and pistachio nuts combined with the perfume of fresh basil. Minestra is Italian for soup. Minestrone is a thick soup that can be made in 20 minutes using bought cooked chicken breasts. Leftover chicken can be used for this recipe. Look for shelled pistachio nuts. They are now available in most supermarkets.

nutty chicken minestrone

2 teaspoons olive oil
50g (2oz) grated carrots
$\frac{1}{2}$ celery stalk, sliced
1 medium tomato, diced
350ml (12fl oz) fat-free, low-sodium chicken stock
350ml (12fl oz) water
225g (8oz) roasted, ready-to-eat chicken strips
Salt and freshly ground black pepper
110g (4oz) washed, ready-to-eat spinach
15g ($\frac{1}{2}$oz) fresh basil
2 tablespoons freshly grated Parmesan cheese
2 tablespoons coarsely chopped pistachio nuts

Heat the oil in a large saucepan on medium-high heat. Add the carrot and celery. Sauté for 5 minutes. Do not brown the vegetables. Stir the vegetables gently, being careful not to break them up. Add the tomato, chicken stock and water. The liquid should cover the vegetables. Add more water, if needed. Bring to a simmer and partially cover with a lid, leaving space for steam to escape. Simmer for 10 minutes. Add the chicken and simmer for 5 more minutes. Add salt and pepper to taste. Remove from heat. Stir in the spinach and basil. Leave to stand for 1 minute. Spoon into 2 soup bowls. Sprinkle each bowl with Parmesan cheese and pistachio nuts. Makes 2 servings.

Per serving: 379 calories, 46.6 grams protein, 10.1 grams carbohydrate, 18.4 grams fat (4.3 saturated), 103 milligrams cholesterol, 731 milligrams sodium, 1.3 grams fibre

spanish tuna-stuffed tomatoes

Olives, pimientos and almonds mix with tuna to make a Spanish tuna salad. This is also a good recipe for leftover chicken or other seafood.

spanish tuna-stuffed tomatoes

2 large tomatoes

2 tablespoons mayonnaise

Freshly ground black pepper

250g (9oz) tinned tuna packed in water, drained

6 stoned green olives, sliced

225g (8oz) sliced sweet pimiento, drained

2 1/2 tablespoons flaked almonds (25g/1oz)

Several lettuce leaves, washed and torn into bite-sized pieces

Cut tomatoes in half, scoop out pulp and seeds, and take a thin slice off the rounded bottom of each half. This will help the tomatoes sit straight on the plate. Set the tomato halves aside. Mix mayonnaise with black pepper to taste. Add the tuna, olives, pimiento and almonds. Mix to combine. Taste for seasoning and add more, if necessary.

Place the lettuce on 2 plates and the tomato halves on the lettuce. Fill the tomatoes with the tuna salad. Serve extra salad on the lettuce. *Makes 2 servings.*

Per serving: 404 calories, 39.2 grams protein, 12.6 grams carbohydrate, 22.5 grams fat (2.3 saturated), 61 milligrams cholesterol, 945 milligrams sodium, 0.2 grams fibre

helpful hints

- *Use good-quality, water-packed, tinned tuna.*
- *To help the tomato halves sit straight, cut a thin slice from the rounded ends.*
- *Any type of lettuce can be used.*

countdown

- *Prepare ingredients.*
- *Make recipe.*

shopping list

FRUIT AND VEG

  2 large tomatoes

  1 small head lettuce

GROCERY

  250g (9oz) tinned tuna packed in water

  1 jar stoned green olives (6 needed)

  1 small jar sweet pimientos

  1 small packet flaked almonds (25g/1oz needed)

STAPLES

  Mayonnaise

  Black peppercorns

helpful hints

- *Any type of lettuce can be used.*

countdown

- *Prepare ingredients.*
- *Assemble salad.*

shopping list

FRUIT AND VEG

1 bag washed, ready-to-eat gourmet salad leaves

1 small bunch spring onions

MEAT

225g (8oz) roasted, ready-to-eat chicken pieces

GROCERY

1 small can sliced water chestnuts

1 jar ground ginger

STAPLES

Olive oil and vinegar dressing

Low-sodium soy sauce

crunchy oriental chicken salad

Roasted or rotisserie chicken takes on a new dimension in this quick salad. Adding ginger and soy sauce to a bottled oil and vinegar dressing gives it an Oriental flavour.

crunchy oriental chicken salad

225g (8oz) roasted, ready-to-eat chicken pieces

175g (6oz) drained, sliced water chestnuts

4 spring onions, sliced

3 tablespoons olive oil and vinegar dressing

2 teaspoons low-sodium soy sauce

1/2 teaspoon ground ginger

150g (5oz) washed, ready-to-eat mixed gourmet salad leaves

Place chicken pieces, water chestnuts and spring onions in a large bowl. Mix dressing, soy sauce and ginger together and pour over chicken. Toss well. Divide salad leaves between 2 plates and spoon chicken salad on top. *Makes 2 servings.*

Per serving: 378 calories, 38.7 grams protein, 17.3 grams carbohydrate, 18.1 grams fat (3.1 saturated), 96 milligrams cholesterol, 437 milligrams sodium, 4.6 grams fibre

crab gratin

Good-quality crabmeat is the secret to this quick lunch. Fresh crabmeat from the seafood counter would be best; but if this is difficult to find, use pasteurised crabmeat.

crab gratin

3 tablespoons mayonnaise
2 tablespoons lemon juice or water
350g (12oz) crabmeat
Salt and freshly ground black pepper
2 large tomatoes, cut into 1cm (¹/₂in) slices
25g (1oz) grated reduced-fat Cheddar cheese

Pre-heat grill. Mix mayonnaise and lemon juice together in a small bowl. Add crabmeat and flake with a fork as it's mixed with the mayonnaise. Add salt and pepper to taste. Place tomato slices on foil-lined baking tray. Spoon crab over tomatoes and sprinkle cheese on top. Place under grill for 2–3 minutes or until cheese melts. Remove to 2 plates and serve.
Makes 2 servings.

Per serving: 382 calories, 37.1 grams protein, 9.1 grams carbohydrate, 21.2 grams fat (4.5 saturated), 149 milligrams cholesterol, 746 milligrams sodium, 0 grams fibre

helpful hints

- *Frozen crab can be used. The flavour will be fine; the crabmeat will be soft.*
- *Pasteurised crabmeat can be found in the refrigerated section of the seafood department.*

countdown

- *Pre-heat grill.*
- *Prepare ingredients.*
- *Make gratin.*

shopping list

FRUIT AND VEG
  2 large tomatoes
DAIRY
  1 small packet grated reduced-fat Cheddar cheese
SEAFOOD
  350g (12oz) crabmeat
STAPLES
  Lemon
  Mayonnaise
  Salt
  Black peppercorns

quick start
dinners

hot pepper prawns

Hot, spicy prawns with lots of garlic are a popular Spanish tapas dish. The prawn dish is normally served on its own for tapas; but by adding a quick salad, it becomes an entire meal. Chicory is a small cigar-shaped head of lettuce that is creamy white. It has tightly packed leaves and can be cleaned by wiping the outer leaves with damp kitchen paper. The leaves will turn brown if soaked in water.

hot pepper prawns

275g (10oz) washed, ready-to-eat spinach
6 garlic cloves, crushed
Salt and freshly ground black pepper
1 tablespoon olive oil
Pinch crushed chilli flakes
350g (12oz) prawns, peeled
2 tablespoons chopped fresh parsley

Place spinach and 3 crushed garlic cloves in a large microwave-safe bowl. Microwave on high for 3 minutes. Add salt and pepper to taste. Toss well. Divide between 2 plates. Heat a medium non-stick frying pan on medium-high heat. Add olive oil and chilli flakes. When oil is hot, add prawns and remaining 3 crushed garlic cloves. Toss prawns in oil for 2–3 minutes or until prawns are no longer translucent. Remove from heat and sprinkle with parsley and salt and pepper to taste. Spoon over spinach including pan juices.
Makes 2 servings.

Per serving: 299 calories, 41.4 grams protein, 11.5 grams carbohydrate, 10.7 grams fat (1.5 saturated), 260 milligrams cholesterol, 426 milligrams sodium, 7.2 grams fibre

red pepper and chicory salad

2 medium heads chicory
1 medium red pepper, sliced into 2.5cm (1in) strips
2 tablespoons olive oil and vinegar dressing
Salt and freshly ground black pepper

Wipe chicory with damp kitchen paper. Cut off about 1cm (½in) from the bottom or flat end and discard. Cut chicory into 1cm (½in) slices and place in a small bowl. Add red pepper strips to bowl. Drizzle with dressing and add salt and pepper to taste. Toss well.
Makes 2 servings.

Per serving: 253 calories, 1.3 grams protein, 7.1 grams carbohydrate, 25.2 grams fat (4.4 saturated), 0 milligrams cholesterol, 239 milligrams sodium, 0 grams fibre

helpful hints

- *Shelled prawns are available at most supermarket seafood counters. The slightly higher cost is worth the time saved.*
- *A quick way to chop parsley is to wash, dry and snip the leaves with scissors right off the stem.*
- *Any type of lettuce can be used for the salad.*

countdown

- *Make salad.*
- *Prepare prawns.*

shopping list

FRUIT AND VEG
1 bag washed, ready-to-eat spinach (275g/10oz needed)
1 medium red pepper
1 small bunch parsley
2 medium heads chicory
SEAFOOD
350g (12oz) shelled prawns
GROCERY
1 small jar crushed chilli flakes
STAPLES
Olive oil
Garlic
Olive oil and vinegar dressing
Salt
Black peppercorns

mediterranean baked fish

Try a taste of the Mediterranean with this baked snapper topped with pinenuts, olives and pimiento. An Italian friend does great courgettes with a hint of melted cheese on top. She told me her secret: grate the courgettes, using a grater with large holes. They cook faster and taste better. I created this quick courgette gratin with memories of her wonderful dish.

mediterranean baked fish

helpful hints

● *Any type of mild white fish fillet can be used in this recipe. Bake about 10 minutes per 2.5cm (1in) of thickness.*
● *Grate the courgettes in a food processor using a julienne cutting blade or use a grater with 0.5cm (¼in) holes.*

countdown

● *Pre-heat oven to 200°C/400°F/gas mark 6.*
● *Make fish.*
● *While fish bakes, make courgettes.*
● *Assemble salad.*

350g (12oz) snapper fillets
Salt and freshly ground black pepper
2 teaspoons olive oil
2 tablespoons pinenuts
6 stoned green olives, cut in half
110g (4oz) sliced sweet pepper, drained

Pre-heat oven to 200°C/400°F/gas mark 6. Line a baking tray with foil. Rinse fish and pat dry with kitchen paper. Sprinkle fish with salt and pepper to taste. Place on prepared baking tray and drizzle oil on top. Bake for 10 minutes. Spoon pinenuts, olives and peppers over fish. Return to oven for 10 minutes.
Makes 2 servings.

Per serving: 255 calories, 33.2 grams protein,
2.2 grams carbohydrate, 8.0 grams fat (1.2 saturated),
62 milligrams cholesterol, 373 milligrams sodium,
0 grams fibre

green salad

150g (5oz) washed, ready-to-eat lettuce
2 tablespoons olive oil and vinegar dressing

Place lettuce in a large bowl and toss with dressing.
Makes 2 servings.

Per serving: 84 calories, 0.6 grams protein,
1.9 grams carbohydrate, 8.5 grams fat (1.3 saturated),
0 milligrams cholesterol, 81 milligrams sodium,
0.3 grams fibre

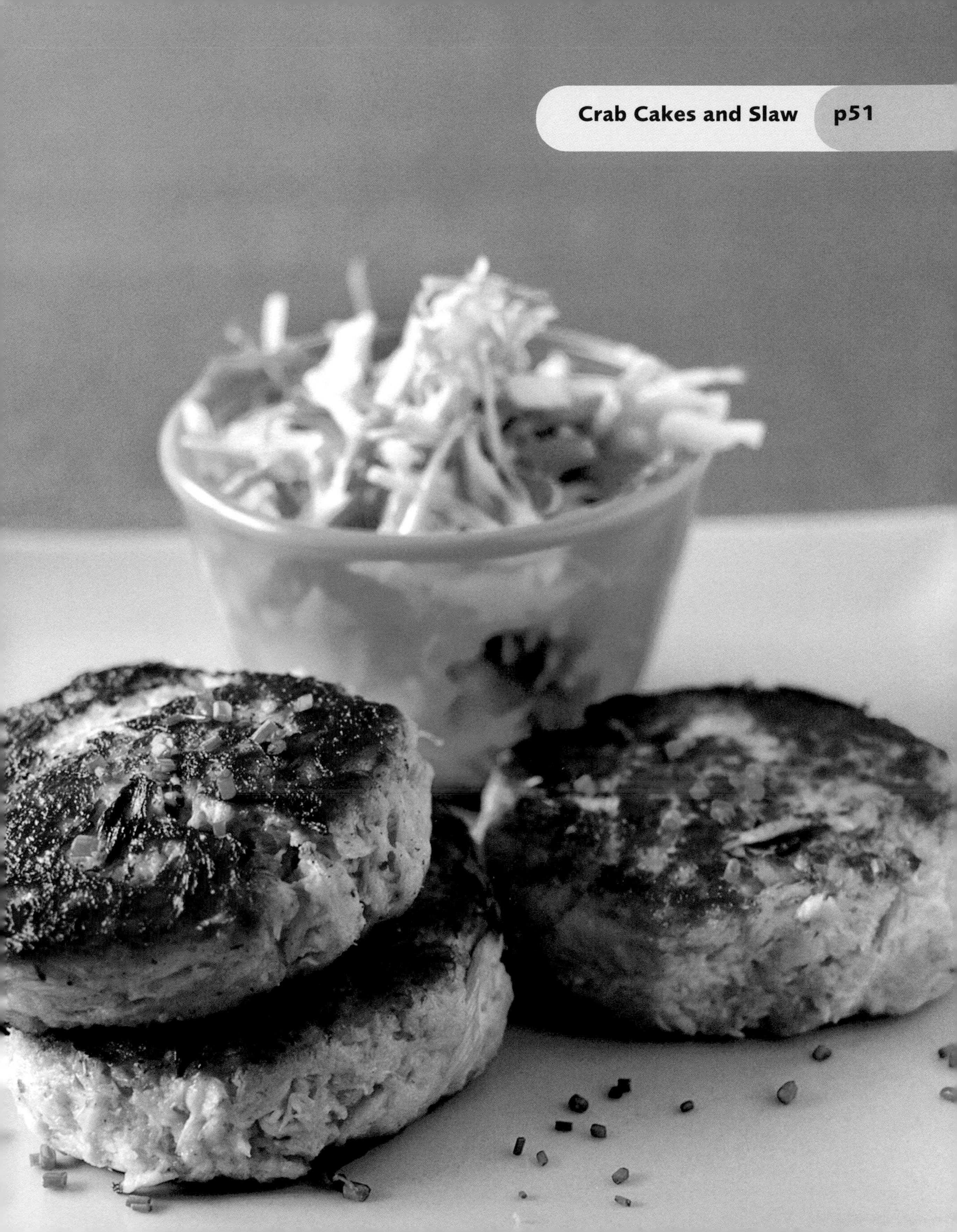

Crab Cakes and Slaw p51

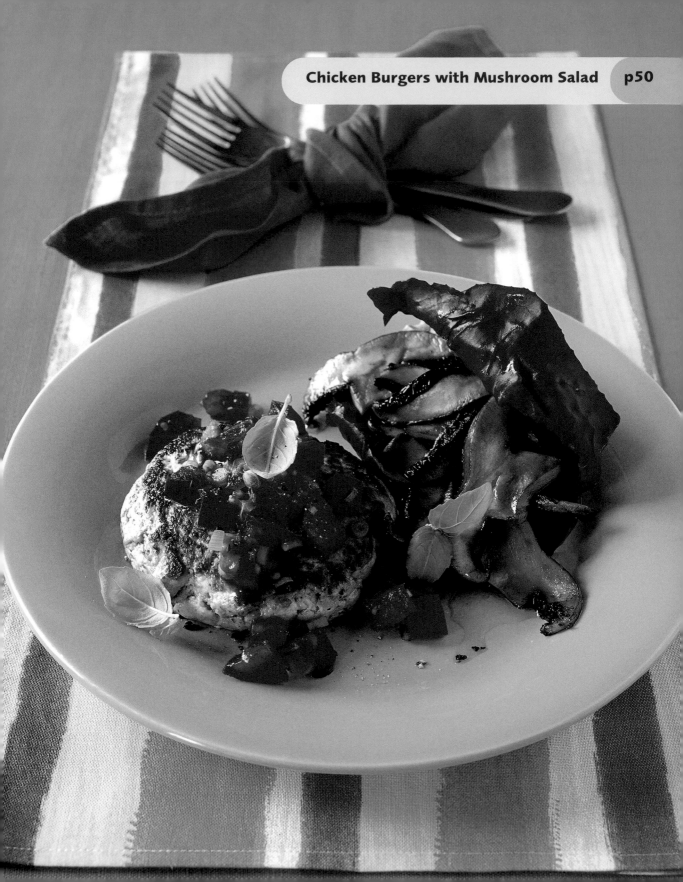

Chicken Burgers with Mushroom Salad **p50**

courgette gratin

450g (1lb) courgettes, grated
2 tablespoons grated Parmesan
cheese
Salt and freshly ground black
pepper
2 teaspoons olive oil

Place courgettes in a microwave-safe bowl. Microwave on high for 2 minutes. If you do not have a microwave oven, bring a small saucepan of water to the boil and add the courgettes. Drain as soon as the water comes back to the boil. Spoon half the courgettes into a shallow ovenproof dish. Sprinkle 1 tablespoon Parmesan cheese and salt and pepper to taste on top. Cover with remaining courgettes and finish with Parmesan cheese and salt and pepper to taste. Drizzle olive oil on top. Place in oven with fish for 5 minutes or until cheese melts.
Makes 2 servings.

Per serving: 129 calories, 7.9 grams protein, 8.0 grams carbohydrate, 8.4 grams fat (2.8 saturated), 9 milligrams cholesterol, 219 milligrams sodium, 1.2 grams fibre

shopping list

FRUIT AND VEG
  450g (1lb) courgettes
  1 bag washed, ready-to-eat
    lettuce
SEAFOOD
  350g (12oz) snapper fillets
GROCERY
  1 small packet pinenuts
    (15g/$\frac{1}{2}$oz needed)
  1 small jar stoned green
    olives
  1 small jar sweet peppers
STAPLES
  Olive oil
  Olive oil and vinegar dressing
  Parmesan cheese
  Salt
  Black peppercorns

helpful hints

- *Parsley or coriander can be used instead of basil in the burgers.*
- *Only 2 tablespoons pesto are needed for the burgers. Extra pesto sauce can be frozen.*
- *To save washing up, cook the mushrooms , then remove and use the same pan for the burgers.*
- *A quick way to chop basil is to wash, dry, then snip the leaves with scissors off the stem.*

countdown

- *Sauté mushrooms and remove from frying pan.*
- *Prepare chicken burgers while mushrooms cook.*
- *Prepare tomato topping for chicken.*
- *Cook chicken burgers.*

shopping list

FRUIT AND VEG
  1 medium tomato
  1 small bunch fresh basil
  1 small bunch spring onions
  225g (8oz) portobello mushrooms
  1 small head radicchio
MEAT
  350g (12oz) chicken mince
GROCERY
  1 small jar prepared pesto sauce
STAPLES
  Olive oil spray
  Garlic
  Olive oil and vinegar dressing
  Salt
  Black peppercorns

chicken burgers with warm mushroom salad

These burgers are tasty and juicy and take only a few minutes to make. Prepared pesto sauce gives the burgers a taste of Italy and keeps the meat juicy.

chicken burgers

350g (12oz) chicken mince
2 tablespoons prepared pesto sauce
$\frac{1}{2}$ teaspoon freshly ground black pepper
Dash of salt
Olive oil spray
1 medium tomato, coarsely chopped
Several basil leaves, cut into bite-sized pieces
1 spring onion, sliced
Salt and freshly ground black pepper

Mix chicken, pesto, black pepper and salt together in a small bowl. Shape into burgers about 9–10cm (3½–4in) in diameter and 1cm (½in) thick. Heat a medium-sized non-stick frying pan on medium-high heat. Spray with olive oil spray and sauté burgers 5 minutes on each side. Remove to 2 dinner plates.
Toss tomato, basil and spring onion together, and add salt and pepper to taste. Spoon over cooked burgers.
Makes 2 servings.

Per serving: 381 calories, 56.6 grams protein, 7.0 grams carbohydrate, 15.0 grams fat (3.9 saturated), 149 milligrams cholesterol, 410 milligrams sodium, 0.8 grams fibre

warm mushroom salad

Olive oil spray
225g (8oz) sliced portobello mushrooms
2 garlic cloves, crushed
Salt and freshly ground black pepper
2 tablespoons olive oil and vinegar dressing
Several radicchio leaves

Heat a non-stick frying pan on medium-high heat and spray with olive oil. Add mushrooms and garlic. Sauté for 5 minutes. Add salt and pepper to taste. Remove to a small bowl. Add dressing and toss well. Place radicchio leaves on 2 dinner plates. Spoon mushrooms on to leaves.
Makes 2 servings.

Per serving: 127 calories, 1.9 grams protein, 5.4 grams carbohydrate, 10.2 grams fat (1.6 saturated), 0 milligrams cholesterol, 80 milligrams sodium, 0.2 grams fibre

crab cakes and slaw

Crab cakes are very popular. Nearly every restaurant seems to have its own version, but the base usually has Worcestershire sauce, hot pepper sauce and onions or spring onions. Fresh crabmeat is best for this recipe. If difficult to find, use pasteurised crabmeat.
Homemade coleslaw is a breeze with a ready-to-eat, sliced coleslaw mix from the fruit and veg department.

crab cakes

450g (1lb) fresh or pasteurised
    crabmeat
2 tablespoons reduced-fat
    mayonnaise
2 tablespoons Worcestershire
    sauce
Several drops hot pepper sauce
4 spring onions, sliced
2 tablespoons Dijon mustard
2 egg whites
3 tablespoons plain breadcrumbs
Salt and freshly ground black
    pepper
2 tablespoons olive oil

Drain crabmeat. Flake meat with a fork while looking for any shell or cartilage that might remain. Mix the mayonnaise, Worcestershire sauce, hot pepper sauce, spring onions, mustard, egg whites and breadcrumbs together in a medium-sized bowl. Add salt and pepper to taste. Stir in crabmeat. Shape into 6 cakes about 7.5cm (3in) in diameter. Heat olive oil in a medium-sized non-stick frying pan on medium heat. Add crab cakes and cook for 5 minutes. Do not move crab cakes during this time. Carefully turn and cook for 5 minutes more. Serve crab cakes with coleslaw.
Makes 2 servings.

Per serving: 435 calories, 46.0 grams protein,
5.5 grams carbohydrate, 22.0 grams fat
(3.4 saturated), 182 milligrams cholesterol,
1572 milligrams sodium, 0 grams fibre

slaw

2 tablespoons reduced-fat
    mayonnaise
1/2 cup distilled white vinegar
Artificial sweetener equivalent to
    2 teaspoons sugar
Salt and freshly ground black
    pepper
225g (8oz) ready-to-eat coleslaw
    mix

Mix mayonnaise, vinegar and artificial sweetener together in a medium-sized bowl. Add salt and pepper to taste. Add coleslaw mix and toss well. Add more salt and pepper, if needed. Place on 2 plates.
Makes 2 servings.

Per serving: 94 calories, 2.0 grams protein,
11.1 grams carbohydrate, 5.4 grams fat
(1.0 saturated), 5 milligrams cholesterol,
139 milligrams sodium, 2.0 grams fibre

helpful hints

● *Frozen crabmeat can be used. The flavour will be fine; the texture will be softer than fresh crabmeat.*
● *Pasteurised crabmeat can be found in the seafood department.*
● *Different types of cabbage, ready-cut, can be found in the fruit and veg section of the supermarket. Use whichever you like.*

countdown

● *Make slaw.*
● *Make crab cakes.*

shopping list

FRUIT AND VEG
    1 pack coleslaw mix
    1 small bunch spring onions
SEAFOOD
    450g (1lb) fresh or
        pasteurised crabmeat
GROCERY
    1 small container plain
        breadcrumbs
STAPLES
    Reduced-fat mayonnaise
    Worcestershire sauce
    Hot pepper sauce
    Dijon mustard
    Eggs (2 needed)
    Olive oil
    Distilled white vinegar
    Artificial sweetener
    Salt
    Black peppercorns

helpful hints

- Any type of green vegetable can be substituted for spinach.
- Look for shelled pistachio nuts in the supermarket.

countdown

- Make spinach and mushrooms.
- Make pork escalopes.

shopping list

FRUIT AND VEG
 2 medium tomatoes
 1 bag washed, ready-to-eat spinach (275g/10oz needed)
 350g (12oz) sliced portobello mushrooms
MEAT
 350g (12oz) pork fillet
GROCERY
 1 small packet shelled pistachio nuts
STAPLES
 Olive oil
 Garlic
 Salt
 Black peppercorns

pork escalopes with spinach and mushrooms

'Pork Escalopes with fresh sautéed tomatoes and garlic,' was the instant answer a famous TV chef gave me when I asked her what she serves her family for a quick meal.

pork escalopes

350g (12oz) pork fillet
2 tablespoons finely chopped pistachio nuts
Salt and freshly ground black pepper
1 teaspoon olive oil
2 medium garlic cloves, crushed
2 medium tomatoes, cut into 2.5cm (1in) pieces

Remove fat from pork and cut into 2.5cm (1in) slices. Place slices between 2 pieces of clingfilm and flatten with the bottom of a heavy pan or a kitchen mallet. Place pistachio nuts on a plate and season with salt and pepper to taste. Press into pork on both sides. Heat oil in a large non-stick frying pan on medium-high heat. Brown pork for 1 minute, then turn and brown second side for 1 minute. Salt and pepper the cooked sides. Remove to a plate. Add garlic and tomatoes to the pan and cook for 3 minutes. Spoon tomatoes over pork and serve.
Makes 2 servings.

Per serving: 398 calories, 53.9 grams protein, 8.8 grams carbohydrate, 16.0 grams fat (3.9 saturated), 159 milligrams cholesterol, 126 milligrams sodium, 0 grams fibre

spinach and mushrooms

275g (10oz) washed, ready-to-eat spinach
350g (12oz) portobello mushrooms, sliced
2 teaspoons olive oil
Salt and freshly ground black pepper

Place spinach and mushrooms in a large microwave-safe bowl. Microwave on high for 5 minutes. Remove and toss well. Add olive oil and salt and pepper to taste. Toss again.
Makes 2 servings.

Per serving: 126 calories, 7.8 grams protein, 11.2 grams carbohydrate, 6.2 grams fat (0.6 saturated), 0 milligrams cholesterol, 174 milligrams sodium, 7.2 grams fibre

roasted salmon and herb sauce

Salmon, sprayed with a little olive oil and salt and pepper, takes on a buttery, creamy texture when roasted in a medium oven for 20 minutes. It is served with a herb sauce that takes only minutes in a food processor.

roasted salmon and herb sauce

2 x 175g (6oz) salmon fillets
Olive oil spray
Salt and freshly ground black pepper
40g (1½oz) rocket
50ml (2fl oz) non-fat natural yoghurt
2 teaspoons fresh lemon or lime juice
1 tablespoon mayonnaise
1 medium tomato, sliced

Pre-heat oven to 180ºC/350ºF/gas mark 4. Line a baking tray with foil. Place salmon on the tray and spray both sides of the fillet with olive oil spray. Sprinkle with salt and pepper to taste. Roast in oven for 20 minutes.

Meanwhile, remove any large stems from the rocket and place in a food processor. Add yoghurt, lemon juice and mayonnaise. Process until smooth. Add salt and pepper to taste. Spoon over roasted salmon. Place sliced tomatoes on the side.

Makes 2 servings.

Per serving: 375 calories, 44.8 grams protein, 6.8 grams carbohydrate, 16.6 grams fat (3.5 saturated), 123 milligrams cholesterol, 180 milligrams sodium, 0 grams fibre

braised asparagus

350g (12oz) asparagus
115ml (4fl oz) water
1 teaspoon olive oil
Salt and freshly ground black pepper

Wash asparagus and cut about 2.5cm (1in) off the woody ends. Place in a large non-stick frying pan just large enough to hold them in one layer. Add the water, olive oil and salt and pepper to taste. Bring to a simmer on medium-high heat and cover with lid. Lower heat to medium-low and cook for 10 minutes. Check the water halfway through the cooking and add more if the pan is dry. Serve with the salmon.

Makes 2 servings.

Per serving: 43 calories, 3 grams protein, 4.5 grams carbohydrate, 206 grams fat (0.4 saturated), 0 milligrams cholesterol, 138 milligrams sodium, 3.6 grams fibre

helpful hints

- *If you do not have a food processor, cut the rocket into small strips and mix with the other ingredients.*
- *If using thin asparagus, cut the braising time in half.*

countdown

- *Pre-heat oven to 180ºC/350ºF/gas mark 4.*
- *Place salmon in oven.*
- *Make asparagus.*
- *While salmon and asparagus cook, make herb sauce.*

shopping list

FRUIT AND VEG
  350g (12oz) asparagus
  1 bunch rocket (40g/1½oz needed)
  1 medium tomato
DAIRY
  1 small pot non-fat natural yoghurt (50ml/2fl oz needed)
SEAFOOD
  2 x 175g (6oz) salmon fillets
STAPLES
  Olive oil
  Olive oil spray
  Lemon
  Mayonnaise
  Salt
  Black peppercorns

tuscan chicken

A fresh tomato-basil relish tops this simple chicken dish. The broccoli takes only minutes to cook in a microwave oven. It's topped with toasted almonds.

tuscan chicken

1 large plum tomato, diced
2 tablespoons diced red onion
50g (2oz) sliced sweet peppers, drained
15g (1/2oz) snipped fresh basil leaves
1/2 tablespoon balsamic vinegar
Salt and freshly ground black pepper
350g (12oz) boneless, skinless chicken breasts
Olive oil spray

Mix tomatoes, onion, sweet peppers and basil together in a small bowl. Add vinegar and toss to mix. Add salt and pepper to taste. Set aside. Place chicken between two pieces of greaseproof paper or foil and flatten with a kitchen mallet or the bottom of a heavy pan to 1cm (1/2in) thick. Heat a large non-stick frying pan on medium-high heat and spray with olive oil spray. Add chicken and sauté 3 minutes per side. Season to taste on the cooked sides. Divide between 2 dinner plates and spoon the tomato relish on top.
Makes 2 servings.

Per serving: 307 calories, 54.6 grams protein, 4.2 grams carbohydrate, 9.0 grams fat (2.1 saturated), 144 milligrams cholesterol, 131 milligrams sodium, 0 grams fibre

helpful hints

- *Any type of ripe tomato can be used for the relish.*
- *Fresh parsley or coriander can be used instead of basil.*
- *A quick way to chop basil is to wash, dry and snip the leaves with scissors off the stem.*
- *To save washing an extra pan, sauté the almonds for a few minutes in a large frying pan, then remove them and use the same pan to cook the chicken.*

countdown

- *Make tomato relish.*
- *Sauté almonds.*
- *Prepare chicken.*
- *Make broccoli..*

toasted almond broccoli

40g (1¹/₂oz) flaked almonds
225g (8oz) broccoli florets
2 teaspoons olive oil
Salt and freshly ground black
  pepper

Heat a non-stick frying pan on medium heat and add the almonds. (This can be done in the same pan to be used for the chicken.) Sauté for 1 minute or until almonds are golden, not brown. Remove and set aside. Place broccoli in a microwave-safe bowl and microwave on high for 4 minutes. Remove and add oil and salt and pepper to taste. Toss well. Sprinkle almonds on top.

Makes 2 servings.

Per serving: 213 calories, 9.7 grams protein, 13.4 grams carbohydrate, 16.2 grams fat (1.4 saturated), 0 milligrams cholesterol, 40 milligrams sodium, 4.9 grams fibre

shopping list

FRUIT AND VEG
  1 large plum tomato
  1 small bunch basil
  225g (8oz) broccoli florets
MEAT
  350g (12oz) boneless,
    skinless chicken breasts
GROCERY
  1 small jar sweet peppers
  40g (1¹/₂oz) flaked almonds
STAPLES
  Red onion
  Olive oil spray
  Olive oil
  Balsamic vinegar
  Salt
  Black peppercorns

which carbs

When I teach classes, I find that this is the most important section. My students are afraid to start reintroducing carbs for fear they will negate all of the benefits they've achieved. Here's how you can prevent gaining lost weight.

The question that keeps coming up at every class is, 'How do I start to add carbohydrates to my meals?' Two things usually happen at this point. You are losing weight and feeling good, so you stay on the Quick Start phase until you get bored or have a special event. Or you think, 'Great. I've lost weight and now I can have the foods I love and forget about the carb restrictions.' But neither solution leads to a healthy lifestyle of low-carb eating.

This section shows you how to start bringing carbs back into your life without gaining weight. I have carefully chosen these recipes to reincorporate high-fibre, low-simple-sugar carbohydrates.

The most important addition in this section is high-fibre cereal in the morning.

As with the other sections, I have organised the menus into a meal-at-a-glance chart incorporating some easy and quick meals from the Super Speed Supper section to accommodate busy mid-week schedules and some more elaborate recipes from the Weekend section suited to a more relaxed weekend pace. They are arranged to give variety throughout the day and over the days of the week.

Breakfast

You can choose from a variety of breakfasts to suit your taste. Quick ideas like microwave Ham-Baked Egg can be done in about 5 minutes. You can also enjoy an Italian Omelette.

Lunch

Cajun Prawn Salad and a quick Horseradish-Crusted Salmon Salad are two of the tempting choices.

Dinner

Five-Spice Tuna Tataki and Veal Piccata are two of the meals that have been carefully planned to slowly reintroduce carbohydrates.

For those days when you are really pressed for time, select Peasant Country Soup and Swordfish in Spanish Sofrito Sauce from the Super Speed Suppers section of the book.

For weekends when you have more time and want something special, try the Steak in Port Wine or Chicken and Walnuts in Lettuce Puffs from the Weekends section of the book.

During the Which Carb 14-Day Meal Plan, which includes the Super Speed Suppers and Weekends meals, you will consume an average of 85–95 grams of carbohydrates per day. Carbohydrate percentage is based on carbohydrates less fibre consumed, which is the normal way of calculating carbohydrate consumption. The balance of these meals is 26 per cent of calories from carbohydrates, 35 per cent of calories from low-fat protein, 24 per cent of calories from mono-unsaturated fat, and 10 per cent of calories from saturated fat.

which carbs 14-day meal plan at a glance

week 1	breakfast	lunch	dinner
sunday	Tomato Frittata 61	Italian Croque Monsieur 69	Crispy Cod with Ratatouille................77
monday	Roast Beef and Cucumber Slices 62	Vietnamese Crab Soup 70	Mediterranean Snapper with Provençal Salad.......................150
tuesday	Sausage Scramble 63	Cajun Prawn Salad 71	Aubergine Parmesan with Linguine...................79
wednesday	Ginger-Cranberry Smoothie with Smoked Ham and Cheese.......................64	Roast Chicken Vegetable Soup 72	Swordfish in Spanish Sofrito Sauce 131
thursday	Ham-Baked Egg 65	Rainbow Tomato Plate 73	Mediterranean Steak 80
friday	Italian Omelette 66	Horseradish-Crusted Salmon Salad..............74	Stir-Fried Veal 82
saturday	New Orleans Prawn Roll 67	Chinese Chicken Salad..........................75	Spiced Cowboy Steak........................149

week 2	breakfast	lunch	dinner
sunday	Tomato Frittata 61	Italian Croque Monsieur...................69	Chicken and Walnuts in Lettuce Puffs............152
monday	Roast Beef and Cucumber Slices 62	Vietnamese Crab Soup 70	Peasant Country Soup 132
tuesday	Sausage Scramble 63	Cajun Prawn Salad 71	Beef Teriyaki with Chinese Noodles..................133
wednesday	Ginger-Cranberry Smoothie with Smoked Ham and Cheese 64	Roast Chicken Vegetable Soup 72	Five-Spice Tuna Tataki 84
thursday	Ham-Baked Egg 65	Rainbow Tomato Plate 73	Chicken with Black Bean Salsa Salad.........86
friday	Italian Omelette........... 66	Horseradish-Crusted Salmon Salad 74	Veal Piccata 88
saturday	New Orleans Prawn Roll.................. 67	Chinese Chicken Salad.........................75	Steak in Port Wine.....................154

which carbs
breakfasts

tomato frittata

Frittatas take about 10 minutes to make. They can be made ahead and eaten at room temperature.

A frittata needs to be cooked on both sides. Some people flip it in the pan. A much easier way is to place it in the oven to finish cooking, under a grill for half a minute, or use this method of covering the frittata with a lid.

tomato frittata

2 whole eggs
6 egg whites
1 medium tomato, cut into 2.5cm (1in) pieces
1 teaspoon dried thyme
50g (2oz) fresh parsley, torn into bite-sized pieces
Salt and freshly ground black pepper
Olive oil spray
6 tablespoons grated semi-skimmed milk mozzarella cheese

Lightly beat whole eggs and egg whites together. Add tomato, thyme, parsley and salt and pepper to taste. Heat a 20–23cm (8–9in) non-stick frying pan over medium heat and spray with olive oil spray. Pour egg mixture into frying pan. Spread to cover pan. Leave to set on the bottom for 1 minute. Sprinkle cheese on top. Turn heat to low, cover with a lid, and leave to cook for 10 minutes or until set. Cut in half and serve on 2 plates.
Makes 2 servings.

bran cereal

225ml (8fl oz) skimmed milk
75g (3oz) high-fibre, no-sugar-added bran cereal

Divide between 2 cereal bowls.
Makes 2 servings.

Per serving: 324 calories, 32.8 grams protein, 36.3 grams carbohydrate, 12.9 grams fat (4.9 saturated), 231 milligrams cholesterol, 575 milligrams sodium, 13.0 grams fibre

helpful hints

● *Dried thyme is used in this recipe. Replace dried herbs after 6 months. If they look grey and old, that's probably how they will taste.*

countdown

● *Start frittata.*
● *While frittata cooks, assemble cereal.*
● *Finish frittata.*

shopping list

FRUIT AND VEG
  1 medium tomato
  1 small bunch parsley
DAIRY
  1 small packet semi-skimmed milk mozzarella cheese
STAPLES
  Dried thyme
  Eggs (8 needed)
  Skimmed milk
  Olive oil spray
  High-fibre, no-sugar-added bran cereal
  Salt
  Black peppercorns

roast beef and cucumber slices

This is a perfect breakfast to eat on the run. The roast beef slices can be made the night before and refrigerated.

helpful hints

● *Try to cut the cucumber slices on the diagonal. Hold the knife at an angle to the cucumber rather than perpendicular to it. This will give more surface area for the roast beef.*

countdown

● *Assemble the roast beef slices.*

● *Assemble cereal.*

shopping list

FRUIT AND VEG
   1 medium cucumber
DELI
   225g (8oz) sliced, lean roast beef
STAPLES
   Skimmed milk
   High-fibre, no-sugar-added bran cereal
   Reduced-fat mayonnaise
   Salt
   Black peppercorns

roast beef and cucumber slices

1 medium cucumber
2 tablespoons reduced-fat mayonnaise
Salt and freshly ground black pepper
225g (8oz) sliced, lean roast beef

Peel cucumber and slice about 0.5cm (¼in) thick on the diagonal. Spread mayonnaise on each slice. Sprinkle with salt and pepper to taste. Fold the sliced roast beef to fit the cucumber slices and place on top. Divide between 2 plates. *Makes 2 servings.*

sausage scramble

Lean, mild turkey sausage makes these scrambled eggs special. If your local butcher makes his own sausages you may be able to get spicy or special herbed versions. Choose whichever you like.

sausage scramble

175g (6oz) mild, low-fat turkey
  sausages, cut into 1cm (1/2in)
  slices
2 whole eggs
4 egg whites
1/2 teaspoon dried oregano
Salt and freshly ground black
  pepper

Heat a medium-sized non-stick frying pan on medium-high heat. Add sausage slices and cook for 3 minutes. While sausage cooks, mix whole eggs and whites together and add oregano and salt and pepper to taste. Add egg mixture to the frying pan. Scramble for 1 minute, or until egg is cooked to desired doneness.
Makes 2 servings.

oatmeal

75g (3oz) oatmeal
450ml (16fl oz) water
225ml (8fl oz) skimmed milk
1 teaspoon cinnamon
Artificial sweetener equivalent to
  2 teaspoons sugar

To prepare in the microwave, combine oatmeal and water together. Microwave on high for 4 minutes. Stir in milk, cinnamon and sweetener. Alternatively, combine oatmeal and water in a small saucepan. Bring to the boil. Cook about 5 minutes over medium heat, stirring occasionally. Stir in milk, cinnamon and sweetener.
Makes 2 servings.

Per serving: 442 calories, 37.3 grams protein,
37.6 grams carbohydrate, 16.9 grams fat
(4.3 saturated), 260 milligrams cholesterol,
777 milligrams sodium, 4.2 grams fibre

helpful hints

● *Dried oregano is used in this recipe. Replace dried herbs after 6 months. If they look grey and old, that's probably how they will taste.*

countdown

● *Make oatmeal.*
● *Make sausage scramble.*

shopping list

MEAT
  175g (6oz) low-fat turkey
    sausages
STAPLES
  Dried oregano
  Eggs (6 needed)
  Oatmeal
  Skimmed milk
  Cinnamon
  Artificial sweetener
  Salt
  Black peppercorns

ginger-cranberry smoothie with smoked ham and cheese

Ginger gives this colourful smoothie an Oriental taste.

ginger-cranberry smoothie

50g (2oz) fresh or frozen cranberries
50ml (2fl oz) water
115ml (4fl oz) non-fat vanilla yoghurt
1 teaspoon ground ginger
Artificial sweetener equivalent to 4 teaspoons sugar
450ml (16fl oz) ice cubes

Place cranberries, water, yoghurt, ginger and sweetener in a blender. Blend until smooth. Add the ice cubes and blend until thick. Pour into 2 glasses.
Makes 2 servings.

smoked ham and cheese

Several lettuce leaves
225g (8oz) smoked, lean ham, cut into 1cm (1/2in) cubes
50g (2oz) reduced-fat Cheddar cheese, torn into bite-sized pieces

Place lettuce on 2 plates with ham and cheese sprinkled on top.
Makes 2 servings.

bran cereal

225ml (8fl oz) skimmed milk
75g (3oz) high-fibre, no-sugar-added bran cereal

Divide between 2 cereal bowls.
Makes 2 servings.

Per serving: 394 calories, 38.4 grams protein, 42.6 grams carbohydrate, 13.1 grams fat (6.2 saturated), 76 milligrams cholesterol, 1473 milligrams sodium, 14.2 grams fibre

ham-baked egg

Baked or shirred eggs are easy to make and are a nice change. They take about 12–15 minutes in the oven. I've shortened the time to 2 minutes by 'baking' them in a microwave oven. The secret is to gently prick the egg yolk in 2 places to break the membrane before placing in the microwave.

ham-baked egg

2 teaspoons olive oil
225g (8oz) lean ham torn into bite-
    sized pieces
2 whole eggs
Salt and freshly ground black
    pepper

Spoon oil into 2 small ramekins. Divide ham into 2 portions and place in the ramekins. Break 1 egg into each dish. With the tip of a very sharp knife make 2 tiny pricks in each egg yolk, just to break the membrane and let steam escape. Sprinkle with salt and pepper to taste. Place one ramekin in a microwave oven. Cover ramekin with a piece of kitchen paper and microwave on high for 1 minute. Remove and serve. Repeat with second ramekin.

Makes 2 servings.

oatmeal

75g (3oz) oatmeal
450ml (16fl oz) water
225ml (8fl oz) skimmed milk
Artificial sweetener equivalent to
    2 teaspoons sugar

To prepare in the microwave, combine oatmeal and water together. Microwave on high for 4 minutes. Stir in milk and sweetener. Alternatively, combine oatmeal and water in a small saucepan. Bring to the boil. Cook about 5 minutes over medium heat, stirring occasionally. Stir in milk and sweetener.

Makes 2 servings.

Per serving: 458 calories, 37.2 grams protein, 35.7 grams carbohydrate, 19.1 grams fat (4.9 saturated), 268 milligrams cholesterol, 1110 milligrams sodium, 4 grams fibre

helpful hints

● *Cook the eggs for 1½ minutes (3 minutes total) for a firmer yolk.*
● *Small dessert or glass bowls can be used instead of ramekins. They should measure about 8–10cm (3–4in) wide and 5cm (2in) deep.*

countdown

● *Assemble eggs and ham in ramekins.*
● *Assemble cereal.*
● *Microwave eggs.*

shopping list

DELI
    225g (8oz) lean, smoked ham
STAPLES
    Eggs (2 needed)
    Skimmed milk
    Olive oil
    Oatmeal
    Salt
    Black peppercorns
    Artificial sweetener

helpful hints

● Buy good-quality Parmesan cheese and grate it yourself or chop it in the food processor. Freeze extra for quick use. You can quickly spoon out what you need and leave the rest frozen.

countdown

● Prepare omelette ingredients.
● Assemble bran cereal.
● Make omelette.

shopping list

DAIRY
  1 small pot ricotta cheese
GROCERY
  1 small jar low-sugar, low-fat chunky marinara sauce
STAPLES
  Egg substitute
  Parmesan cheese
  Skimmed milk
  Olive oil
  High-fibre, no-sugar-added bran cereal
  Black peppercorns

italian omelette

A perfect omelette is golden on the top with a delicate creamy centre. The secret is to cook it over medium-high heat for only a couple of minutes while gently scraping the side to make sure all of the egg is cooked.

italian omelette

50g (2oz) ricotta cheese
50ml (2fl oz) bottled low-sugar, low-fat chunky marinara sauce
15g (½oz) grated Parmesan cheese
350ml (12fl oz) egg substitute
Freshly ground black pepper
2 teaspoons olive oil

Mix ricotta cheese, marinara sauce and Parmesan cheese together and set aside. Mix egg substitute with pepper to taste. Heat oil in a medium-sized non-stick frying pan on medium-high heat. Pour in the egg mixture. Let the eggs set for about 30 seconds. Tip the pan and lightly move the eggs so that they all set. Spread the cheese mixture on half the omelette and fold the omelette in half. Slide out of the pan by tipping the pan and holding a plate vertically against the side of the pan. Turn the pan and plate to invert the omelette on to the plate. Cut in half and serve on 2 plates.
Makes 2 servings.

bran cereal

225ml (8fl oz) skimmed milk
75g (3oz) high-fibre, no-sugar-added bran cereal

Divide between 2 cereal bowls.
Makes 2 servings.

365 calories, 32.6 grams protein, 36.8 grams carbohydrate, 12.4 grams fat (4.5 saturated), 17 milligrams cholesterol, 1076 milligrams sodium, 13.0 grams fibre

new orleans prawn roll

Prawns and hot pepper sauce give this roll-up a hint of New Orleans cooking. The egg is cooked like a crêpe and used as a wrap.

new orleans prawn roll

225g (8oz) cooked prawns, peeled and deveined
2 tablespoons mayonnaise
Several drops hot pepper sauce
Salt and freshly ground black pepper
225ml (8fl oz) egg substitute
Olive oil spray

Coarsely chop the prawns. Add mayonnaise and hot pepper sauce. Add salt and pepper to taste. Mix egg substitute with salt and pepper to taste. Heat a medium-sized non-stick frying pan on medium-high heat. Spray with olive oil spray and pour half the egg substitute into the pan and spread to make a thin layer. Leave to cook for 2 minutes. Turn over for 1 minute. Remove from heat. Spread half the prawn mixture on top. Roll up and place on a plate. Repeat for second serving.
Makes 2 servings.

oatmeal

225ml (8fl oz) oatmeal
450ml (16fl oz) water
225ml (8fl oz) skimmed milk
Artificial sweetener equivalent to 2 teaspoons sugar

To prepare in the microwave, combine oatmeal and water together. Microwave on high for 4 minutes. Stir in milk and sweetener. Alternatively, combine oatmeal and water in a small saucepan. Bring to the boil. Cook for about 5 minutes over medium heat, stirring occasionally. Stir in milk and sweetener.
Makes 2 servings.

Per serving: 473 calories, 44.3 grams protein, 36.5 grams carbohydrate, 16.0 grams fat (2.6 saturated), 180 milligrams cholesterol, 535 milligrams sodium, 4 grams fibre

helpful hints

● *Cooked, shelled prawns can be found in the fish department or frozen in most supermarkets.*
● *Use the pulse button on a food processor to coarsely chop the prawns.*

countdown

● *Prepare prawn filling.*
● *Make prawn roll.*
● *Assemble cereal.*

shopping list

SEAFOOD
 225g (8oz) cooked, peeled, deveined prawns
STAPLES
 Mayonnaise
 Egg substitute
 Olive oil spray
 Hot pepper sauce
 Skimmed milk
 Oatmeal
 Artificial sweetener
 Salt
 Black peppercorns

which carbs
lunches

italian croque monsieur

Nearly every brasserie in Paris serves a version of croque monsieur (grilled ham and cheese sandwich). Here is an Italian version.

italian croque monsieur

Olive oil spray

4 slices wholemeal bread

110g (4oz) semi-skimmed milk mozzarella cheese, sliced

225g (8oz) lean ham, sliced

1 medium tomato, sliced

25g (1oz) fresh basil, torn into bite-sized pieces (optional)

Place salmon on a cutting board. Soften cream Pre-heat grill. Line a baking tray with foil and spray with olive oil spray. Place bread on foil and spray bread. Place cheese and then ham on bread. Top with sliced tomato. Grill for 2 minutes or until cheese melts. Remove and sprinkle with basil.

Makes 2 servings.

Per serving: 424 calories, 44.7 grams protein, 26.3 grams carbohydrate, 18.9 grams fat (8.3 saturated), 86 milligrams cholesterol, 1483 milligrams sodium, 6.0 grams fibre

dessert

275g (10oz) watermelon cubes

Divide between 2 small dessert dishes.

Makes 2 servings.

Per serving: 49 calories, 1.0 gram protein, 11.0 grams carbohydrate, 0.6 grams fat (0.1 saturated), 0 milligrams cholesterol, 3 milligrams sodium, 0.8 grams fibre

helpful hints

● *Watermelon cubes can be found in the fruit and veg section of some supermarkets.*

countdown

● *Pre-heat grill.*
● *Make sandwich.*
● *While sandwich toasts, place watermelon in dishes.*

shopping list

FRUIT AND VEG

1 small bunch basil

1 medium tomato

1 small container watermelon cubes

DAIRY

1 small packet semi-skimmed milk mozzarella cheese

DELI

225g (8oz) lean ham

STAPLES

Olive oil spray

Wholemeal bread

vietnamese crab soup

This soup is filled with the fragrant flavours of South-east Asia. As with most Asian dishes, it takes a little longer to prepare the ingredients, but then it takes less than 5 minutes to cook. Lemongrass, which adds a special lemon flavour to Asian dishes, can be found in some supermarkets. It looks a bit like a spring onion, but the stalks are a pale green colour, hard and dry. Use the white bulbous end for the soup.

helpful hints

- If fresh crab is unavailable, use crab, or prawns.
- One tablespoon lime juice can be substituted for the lemongrass.
- A quick way to chop ginger is to peel, cut into chunks, and press through a garlic press with large holes. The ginger pulp will not go through a small garlic press. Just the juice is enough to flavour the dish.
- Cubed fresh honeydew melon can be found in the fruit and veg section of most supermarkets.

countdown

- Assemble ingredients for soup.
- Place melon cubes in dessert dishes.
- Complete soup.

shopping list

FRUIT AND VEG
   1 small bunch lemongrass
      (2 stalks needed)
   1 lime
   150g (5oz) fresh mange tout
   1 small bag bean sprouts
   1 small bunch spring onions
   1 small container fresh
      honeydew melon cubes
   1 small piece fresh ginger
SEAFOOD
   350g (12oz) fresh or
      pasteurised crabmeat
GROCERY
   1 small bottle sesame oil
STAPLES
   Fat-free, low-sodium chicken
      stock
   Hot pepper sauce
   Salt
   Black peppercorns

vietnamese crab soup

450ml (16fl oz) fat-free, low-sodium chicken stock
450ml (16fl oz) water
2 stalks lemongrass, tender white base only, sliced
1 tablespoon peeled and coarsely chopped fresh ginger
1 tablespoon lime zest
150g (5oz) fresh mange tout, trimmed
75g (3oz) bean sprouts
350g (12oz) fresh or pasteurised crabmeat, drained
2 tablespoons sesame oil
Several drops hot pepper sauce
Salt and freshly ground black pepper
2 spring onions, sliced

Place chicken stock and water in a large saucepan. Add lemongrass, ginger, lime zest and mange tout. Bring to a simmer on medium heat and cook for 2 minutes. Add bean sprouts and crab. Simmer for 2 more minutes. Remove from heat and add hot pepper sauce, sesame oil and salt and pepper to taste. Ladle into 2 soup bowls and sprinkle spring onions on top.
Makes 2 servings.

Per serving: 343 calories, 37.3 grams protein, 11.8 grams carbohydrate, 15.8 grams fat (2.2 saturated), 133 milligrams cholesterol, 1070 milligrams sodium, 2.6 grams fibre

dessert

275g (10oz) honeydew melon cubes

Divide between 2 small dessert plates.
Makes 2 servings.

Per serving: 57 calories, 1.4 grams protein, 13.4 grams carbohydrate, 0.4 grams fat (0 saturated), 0 milligrams cholesterol, 14 milligrams sodium, 0.5 grams fibre

cajun prawn salad

The hot spices of Louisiana Cajun country flavour this quick prawn salad.

cajun prawn salad

2 tablespoons no-sugar-added oil
  and vinegar dressing
2 garlic cloves, crushed
½ teaspoon cayenne
1 teaspoon dried oregano
1 teaspoon dried thyme
350g (12oz) cooked prawns,
  peeled, deveined and cut in half
1 small head cos lettuce heart
1 medium red pepper, cut into
  small cubes

In a small bowl, mix dressing with garlic, cayenne, oregano and thyme. Add prawns and toss well. Tear lettuce into bite-sized pieces and place on 2 plates. Mix red pepper with prawns and spoon prawns and dressing over lettuce.
Makes 2 servings.

Per serving: 301 calories, 37.2 grams protein, 10.6 grams carbohydrate, 11.7 grams fat (1.9 saturated), 260 milligrams cholesterol, 342 milligrams sodium, 0.9 grams fibre

dessert

2 oranges

Divide between 2 small plates.
Makes 2 servings.

Per serving: 62 calories, 1.2 grams protein, 15.4 grams carbohydrate, 0.2 grams fat (0 saturated), 0 milligrams cholesterol, 0 milligrams sodium, 3.1 grams fibre

helpful hints

● *Cooked, shelled prawns can be found in the fish department or frozen in the frozen section of most supermarkets.*

● *Prepared Cajun spice mix can be used instead of the spice mixture in the recipe. Make sure no sugar or salt is added to the mixture.*

● *Dried oregano, thyme and cayenne pepper are used in this recipe. Replace dried herbs after 6 months. If they look grey and old, that's probably how they will taste.*

countdown

● *Make dressing.*
● *Complete salad.*

shopping list

FRUIT AND VEG
  1 small head cos lettuce heart
  1 medium red pepper
  2 oranges
SEAFOOD
  350g (12oz) cooked, peeled and deveined prawns
STAPLES
  Dried thyme
  Dried oregano
  Cayenne pepper
  No-sugar-added oil and vinegar dressing
  Garlic

roast chicken vegetable soup

A cheery bowl of soup is a treat any time of year. This soup uses roasted, ready-to-eat chicken and can be ready in less than 15 minutes. The soup tastes great the second day. Make extra if you have time and save for a second day or freeze.

helpful hints

- *Any type of mushroom can be used.*
- *Buy good-quality Parmesan cheese and grate it yourself or chop it in the food processor. Freeze extra for quick use. You can quickly spoon out what you need and leave the rest frozen.*
- *Fresh pineapple cubes can be found in the fruit and veg section of most supermarkets.*

countdown

- *Start soup.*
- *While soup cooks, assemble pineapple dessert.*
- *Complete soup.*

shopping list

FRUIT AND VEG
  225g (8oz) mushrooms
  1 small bunch thyme or dried thyme
  1 small container fresh pineapple cubes
MEAT
  225g (8oz) roasted, ready-to-eat chicken pieces
STAPLES
  Yellow onion
  Celery
  Fat-free, low-sodium chicken stock
  Parmesan cheese
  Olive oil
  Salt
  Black peppercorns

roast chicken vegetable soup

2 teaspoons olive oil
110g (4oz) sliced yellow onion
1 celery stalk, sliced
225g (8oz) mushrooms, sliced
450ml (16fl oz) fat-free, low-sodium chicken stock
225ml (8fl oz) water
2 large sprigs fresh thyme or 1 teaspoon dried thyme
225g (8oz) roasted, ready-to-eat chicken pieces
Salt and freshly ground black pepper
2 tablespoons grated Parmesan cheese

Heat oil in a large saucepan over medium-high heat and add onion and celery. Sauté for 3 minutes. Add mushrooms, stock, water and thyme. Reduce heat to medium and simmer for 7 minutes. Add chicken and cook for 2 minutes or until chicken is warmed through. Remove thyme sprigs and add salt and pepper to taste. Spoon into 2 soup bowls and sprinkle Parmesan on top.
Makes 2 servings.

Per serving: 334 calories, 44.8 grams protein, 8.3 grams carbohydrate, 13.5 grams fat (3.6 saturated), 103 milligrams cholesterol, 858 milligrams sodium, 0.5 grams fibre

dessert

275g (10oz) pineapple cubes

Divide between 2 dessert dishes.
Makes 2 servings.

Per serving: 77 calories, 0.6 grams protein, 19.2 grams carbohydrate, 0.7 grams fat (0 saturated), 0 milligrams cholesterol, 1 milligram sodium, 2.4 grams fibre

rainbow tomato plate

This colourful salad plate accented with red and yellow tomatoes takes only 5 minutes to assemble.

rainbow tomato plate

2 small red tomatoes, sliced
2 small yellow tomatoes, sliced
*1 medium cucumber, peeled and
    sliced*
25g (1oz) pinenuts
*175g (6oz) smoked chicken
    breast, cut into cubes*
*2 tablespoons no-sugar-added oil
    and vinegar dressing*
*Salt and freshly ground black
    pepper*

Arrange the sliced tomatoes and cucumber in circles on 2 plates, alternating red tomato slices, yellow tomato slices and cucumber slices. The slices should cover the plate. Sprinkle chicken cubes and pinenuts over tomatoes. Drizzle dressing over the top. Sprinkle with salt and pepper to taste.
Makes 2 servings.

Per serving: 354 calories, 32.1 grams protein, 15.1 grams carbohydrate, 13.0 grams fat (2.2 saturated), 72 milligrams cholesterol, 161 milligrams sodium, 0.9 grams fibre

dessert

225ml (8fl oz) non-fat fruit yoghurt

Divide yoghurt between 2 small dessert bowls.
Makes 2 servings.

Per serving: 70 calories, 5.5 grams protein, 11.5 grams carbohydrate, 0 grams fat (0 saturated), 3 milligrams cholesterol, 95 milligrams sodium, 0 grams fibre

helpful hints

- *Any type of tomatoes can be used.*
- *Any flavour non-fat yoghurt can be used for dessert.*
- *Extra pinenuts can be stored in the freezer.*

countdown

- *Make salad plate.*
- *Serve yoghurt.*

shopping list

FRUIT AND VEG
  2 small red tomatoes
  2 small yellow tomatoes
  1 medium cucumber
DAIRY
  1 pot non-fat fruit yoghurt
DELI
  *175g (6oz) smoked chicken
    breast*
GROCERY
  1 small packet pinenuts
STAPLES
  *No-sugar-added oil and
    vinegar dressing*
  Salt
  Black peppercorns

horseradish-crusted salmon salad

A spicy, creamy crust covers the rich salmon fillet for this quick lunch. The salmon tastes great served either hot or at room temperature.

helpful hints

- *The salmon keeps well and can be served the next day. Make double the portion for another quick lunch.*

countdown

- *Pre-heat grill.*
- *Make salmon.*
- *While salmon cooks, prepare lettuce and cucumber.*

shopping list

FRUIT AND VEG

1 bag washed, ready-to-eat cos lettuce leaves

1 medium cucumber

2 medium apples

SEAFOOD

225g (8oz) salmon fillet

GROCERY

1 small jar prepared horseradish

STAPLES

Olive oil spray

Mayonnaise

Salt

Black peppercorns

horseradish-crusted salmon salad

Olive oil spray

225g (8oz) salmon fillet

Salt and freshly ground black pepper

2 tablespoons prepared horseradish

2 tablespoons mayonnaise

150g (5oz) washed, ready-to-eat cos lettuce leaves

1 medium cucumber, peeled and sliced

Pre-heat grill. Line a baking tray with foil and spray with olive oil spray. Place salmon on the tray. Sprinkle with salt and pepper to taste. Grill for 3 minutes. Mix horseradish and mayonnaise together. Remove salmon and turn over. Spread with horseradish mixture. Return to grill for 3 minutes. Place lettuce and cucumber on 2 plates. Remove salmon and divide in half. Place over salad.

Makes 2 servings.

> Per serving: 340 calories, 30.4 grams protein, 8.7 grams carbohydrate, 19.3 grams fat (3.4 saturated), 85 milligrams cholesterol, 181 milligrams sodium, 1.5 grams fibre

dessert

2 medium apples

Serve 1 apple per person.

Makes 2 servings.

> Per serving: 81 calories, 0.3 grams protein, 21.1 grams carbohydrate, 0.5 grams fat (0.1 saturated), 0 milligrams cholesterol, 0 milligrams sodium, 3.7 grams fibre

chinese chicken salad

Adding Chinese five-spice powder and soy sauce to a bottled oil and vinegar dressing gives this salad an aromatic Chinese flavour.

chinese chicken salad

1 tablespoon low-sodium soy sauce

½ teaspoon five-spice powder

2 tablespoons no-sugar-added oil and vinegar dressing

75g (3oz) bean sprouts

225g (8oz) roasted, ready-to-eat chicken pieces

Salt and freshly ground black pepper

175g (6oz) sliced Chinese cabbage

4 clementines, peeled and segmented

In a medium-sized bowl, mix soy sauce, five-spice powder and dressing together. Add the bean sprouts and chicken and toss well. Add salt and pepper to taste. Place cabbage on 2 plates and spoon chicken mixture on top. Sprinkle clementine segments on top.

Makes 2 servings.

Per serving: 388 calories, 40.6 grams protein, 28.9 grams carbohydrate, 14.5 grams fat (2.5 saturated), 96 milligrams cholesterol, 485 milligrams sodium, 2.4 grams fibre

helpful hints

- *Chinese cabbage is also called Chinese leaves.*
- *Any type of lettuce can be used.*

countdown

- *Mix dressing ingredients together.*
- *Complete salad.*
- *Assemble dessert.*

shopping list

FRUIT AND VEG

1 small Chinese cabbage (Chinese leaves)

1 small packet fresh bean sprouts

4 clementines

MEAT

225g (8oz) roasted, ready-to-eat chicken pieces

GROCERY

1 small jar five-spice powder

STAPLES

Low-sodium soy sauce

No-sugar-added oil and vinegar dressing

Salt

Black peppercorns

which carbs
dinners

crispy cod with ratatouille

For this quick meal, freshly made ratatouille, a tasty blend of Provençal vegetables, is combined with juicy fish fillets. Coating the fish fillet with polenta gives it a crispy crust without having to deep-fry it.

I am often asked how to cook fish so that it's juicy and not dried out. The general rule is to cook fish for 10 minutes for each 2.5cm (1in) of thickness. If the fish is thicker, cook it a little longer, or if thinner, cook it a shorter time.

crispy cod

350g (12oz) cod fillet
2 tablespoons polenta
Salt and freshly ground black
    pepper
2 teaspoons olive oil

Wash fish fillet and pat dry with kitchen paper. Season polenta with salt and pepper to taste. Dip fish into polenta, making sure both sides are well coated. Heat olive oil in a medium-sized non-stick frying pan on medium-high heat. Add fish and sauté for 5 minutes. Turn and sauté another 5 minutes for a 2.5cm (1in) thick fillet. Reduce cooking time to 8 total minutes for 1cm (½in) fillet. Divide in half and serve.
Makes 2 servings.

> Per serving: 203 calories, 29.3 grams protein, 5.6 grams carbohydrate, 6.0 grams fat (1.0 saturated), 116 milligrams cholesterol, 136 milligrams sodium, 0 grams fibre

ratatouille

175g (6oz) aubergine, washed and
    sliced
175g (6oz) courgettes, washed
    and sliced
110g (4oz) sliced red onion
2 medium garlic cloves, crushed
450ml (16fl oz) low-sodium, low-
    sugar tomato or pasta sauce
115ml (4fl oz) water
2 teaspoons olive oil
Salt and freshly ground black
    pepper

Add aubergine, courgettes, onion, garlic, tomato sauce and water to a medium-sized saucepan. Bring to a simmer over medium-high heat. Lower heat and cover. Simmer for 15 minutes. Vegetables should be cooked through but a little firm. Stir in olive oil and add salt and pepper to taste.
Makes 2 servings.

> Per serving: 223 calories, 5.9 grams protein, 18.9 grams carbohydrate, 4.7 grams fat (0.6 saturated), 0 milligrams cholesterol, 44 milligrams sodium, 3.5 grams fibre

helpful hints

- You can use haddock or bass in place of cod.
- For the pumpkin pudding, use the mixture of spices given or use a mixed spice mixture, making sure no sugar has been added.

countdown

- Start ratatouille.
- Make pumpkin pudding.
- Prepare fish.

crispy cod with ratatouille continued

shopping list

FRUIT AND VEG

   175g (6oz) aubergine

   175g (6oz) courgettes

DAIRY

   1 pot non-fat vanilla yoghurt

SEAFOOD

   350g (12oz) cod fillets

GROCERY

   1 small packet polenta

   1 small tin 100% pure pumpkin

   1 small packet pecan pieces

STAPLES:

   Red onion

   Garlic

   Olive oil

   *Low-sodium, low-sugar
     tomato or pasta sauce*

   Artificial sweetener

   Ground cinnamon

   Grated nutmeg

   Salt

   Black peppercorns

pumpkin pudding

*175ml (6fl oz) tinned 100% pure
   pumpkin*

*175ml (6fl oz) non-fat vanilla
   yoghurt*

⅛ teaspoon ground cinnamon

⅛ teaspoon grated nutmeg

*Artificial sweetener equivalent to
   2 teaspoons sugar*

2 tablespoons pecan pieces

Mix together pumpkin, cinnamon, nutmeg and sweetener. Fold into yoghurt. Toast pecan pieces in the oven or under a grill until golden, about 2 minutes. Divide pumpkin mixture between 2 small dessert bowls or ramekins and sprinkle pecans on top.

Makes 2 servings.

Per serving: 162 calories, 6.2 grams protein, 18.4 grams carbohydrate, 8.4 grams fat (0.9 saturated), 2 milligrams cholesterol, 73 milligrams sodium, 3.7 grams fibre

aubergine parmesan with linguine

Aubergine parmesan, my husband's favourite dish, is a Neapolitan dish made with slices of fried aubergine baked in a rich tomato sauce and Parmesan cheese. I've created this quick version by microwaving the slices instead. It also makes the dish much lighter, as fried aubergine soaks up a lot of oil during the cooking.

aubergine parmesan with linguine

Olive oil spray

225g (8oz) aubergine, cut into 0.5cm (¼in) slices

Salt and freshly ground black pepper

350ml (12fl oz) low-sodium, no-sugar-added, tomato sauce

175g (6oz) lean minced beef

40g (1½oz) rocket leaves

110g (4oz) low-fat ricotta cheese

3 tablespoons water

3 tablespoons grated Parmesan cheese

50g (2oz) wholemeal linguine

2 teaspoons olive oil

Pre-heat the grill. Bring a large saucepan filled with 3–4 litres (5–7 pints) of water to the boil. Arrange aubergine slices on a 23–25cm (9–10in) microwave-safe pie dish. Spray with olive oil spray and sprinkle with salt and pepper to taste. Cover with clingfilm or a plate. Microwave on high for 3 minutes. Carefully remove cover. Remove aubergine to a plate and set aside.

Mix tomato sauce and minced beef together in a microwave-safe bowl. Microwave on high for 3 minutes. Spoon a layer of meat sauce into the bottom of the pie dish. Place rocket leaves over sauce. Place a layer of aubergine slices over the sauce and sprinkle with a little salt and pepper to taste. Repeat with the sauce, aubergine and salt and pepper. Mix ricotta cheese with water to form a sauce consistency. Add more water if necessary. Spoon ricotta cheese over top of aubergine dish. Sprinkle with Parmesan cheese. Grill for 5 minutes until sauce is bubbly and cheese melted. Place linguine in boiling water for 9 minutes. Drain and toss with olive oil and add salt and pepper to taste.

Place linguine on 2 dinner plates and serve aubergine parmesan on top.

Makes 2 servings.

Per serving: 597 calories, 53.3 grams protein, 50.1 grams carbohydrate, 19.1 grams fat (10.1 saturated), 122 milligrams cholesterol, 446 milligrams sodium, 9.1 grams fibre

helpful hints

● *Buy Parmesan cheese and grate it yourself or chop it in a food processor. Freeze extra for quick use. You can spoon out what you need and leave the rest frozen.*

● *This dish can be prepared and assembled in advance and refrigerated several hours or overnight. Bring to room temperature and grill as needed.*

countdown

● *Pre-heat grill.*
● *Boil water for pasta.*
● *Microwave aubergine.*
● *Mix ricotta.*
● *Assemble aubergine parmesan and place under grill.*
● *Boil linguine.*

shopping list

FRUIT AND VEG
  225g (8oz) aubergine
  1 small bunch rocket
DAIRY
  1 small pot low-fat ricotta cheese
MEAT
  175g (6oz) lean minced beef
GROCERY
  1 small packet wholemeal linguine (50g/2oz needed)
STAPLES
  Parmesan cheese
  Olive oil
  Low-sodium, no-sugar-added tomato sauce (350ml/12fl oz needed)
  Salt
  Black peppercorns

mediterranean steak

Sautéed steak flavoured with the bountiful produce of the Mediterranean provides a quick, 15-minute dinner.

Pre-cooked, packaged couscous takes only 5 minutes to make. It's made from semolina flour and is in fact a form of pasta rather than a grain as many people think. You just boil water, remove from heat, add the couscous, cover, and leave to stand. For this dinner, I've added fresh mint and chopped tomatoes to add a fresh flavour that goes well with the steak.

mediterranean steak

350g (12oz) steak (sirloin or fillet)
½ teaspoon cayenne pepper
Olive oil spray
3 tablespoons sliced pimiento-stuffed green olives
2 tablespoons capers
Salt and freshly ground black pepper

Remove fat from steak and sprinkle both sides with cayenne. Heat a small, non-stick frying pan over medium-high heat. Spray with olive oil spray. Brown steak for 2 minutes per side. Sprinkle olives and capers into frying pan and over steak. Lower heat to medium and cook 2 minutes for medium-rare. Cook 2 minutes longer for thick steak. Add salt and pepper to taste.

To serve, place couscous on 2 dinner plates, carve steak and place on top. Spoon any pan juices over steak.
Makes 2 servings.

Per serving: 356 calories, 55.8 grams protein, 0.3 grams carbohydrate, 16.4 grams fat (7.1 saturated), 140 milligrams cholesterol, 548 milligrams sodium, 0 grams fibre

minted couscous

115ml (4fl oz) water
50g (2oz) couscous
1 small tomato, diced
½ cucumber, cut into cubes
15g (½ oz) chopped fresh mint
Salt and freshly ground black pepper

Bring water to the boil. Remove from heat and add couscous, tomatoes and cucumber. Cover with a lid and leave to stand for 5 minutes. When ready, fluff with a fork. Add mint and salt and pepper to taste.
Makes 2 servings.

Per serving: 144 calories, 5.9 grams protein, 30.0 grams carbohydrate, 0.9 grams fat (0 saturated), 0 milligrams cholesterol, 11 milligrams sodium, 1.9 grams fibre

helpful hints

- *Use a frying pan that just fits the steak to capture the pan juices. A larger pan will cause the juices to boil away.*
- *Buy sliced olives.*

countdown

- *Bring water for couscous to the boil.*
- *Prepare ingredients for steak.*
- *Make couscous.*
- *Finish steak.*

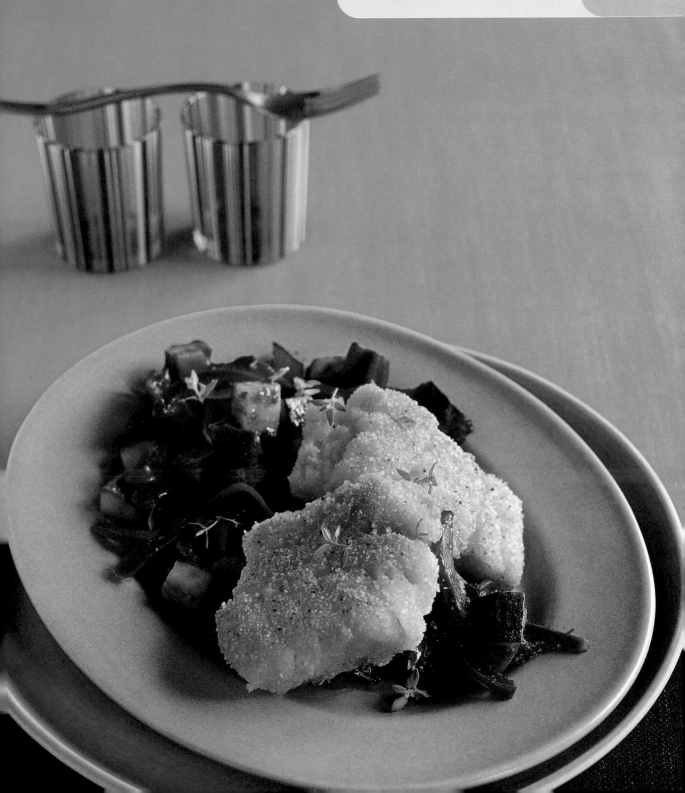

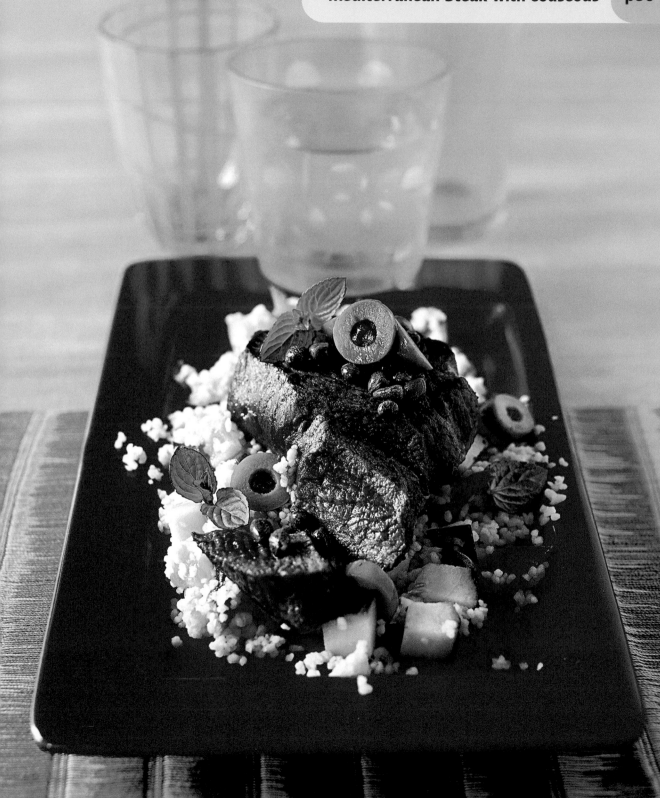
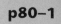

spiced peaches

*2 medium peaches, stoned and
  sliced*
1 teaspoon ground cinnamon
1 teaspoon allspice
*Artificial sweetener equivalent to
  1 teaspoon sugar*
2 sprigs fresh mint

Arrange peach slices in a circle on 2 small
dessert plates. Mix cinnamon, allspice and
sweetener together. Sprinkle mixture over
peach slices. Place both dishes in a microwave
oven on high for 1 minute. Remove, garnish
with mint leaves, and serve.
Makes 2 servings.

Per serving: 39 calories, 0.6 grams protein, 10.7 grams
carbohydrate, 0.1 gram fat (0 saturated), 0 milligrams
cholesterol, 0 milligrams sodium, 0.5 grams fibre

shopping list

FRUIT AND VEG
  1 small bunch fresh mint
  1 small tomato
  2 medium peaches
  ½ cucumber
MEAT
  *350g (12oz) steak (sirloin
    or fillet)*
GROCERY
  1 small packet couscous
  *1 small jar/can pimiento-
    stuffed green olives*
  1 small jar capers
  1 small jar allspice
STAPLES
  Olive oil spray
  Cayenne pepper
  Ground cinnamon
  Artificial sweetener
  Salt
  Black peppercorns

stir-fried veal

A stir-fry dish with a mystery flavour makes a delicious, quick dinner. The grapefruit nearly melts away leaving an intriguing flavour and texture.

Stir-fry dishes take a little extra time to prepare the ingredients, but take only a few minutes to cook. I find it is best to line up all of the stir-fry ingredients on a plate or chopping board in order of use. You won't have to keep referring to the recipe while cooking.

Brown rice takes about 45 minutes to cook. There are several brands of quick-cooking brown rice available. Their cooking time ranges from 10 to 30 minutes. I find the 30-minute rice has more flavour, but any quick-cooking brown rice will work for this dinner.

helpful hints

- Your wok or frying pan should be very hot so the veal will be crisp, not steamed.
- Peel and segment grapefruit over a bowl to catch the juice. This will give you the 2 tablespoons of grapefruit juice needed for the recipe.
- The grapefruit segments should be about the same size as the veal. If they are too large, cut them in half.
- Bought grapefruit segments can be used. Make sure they are natural, without added sugar.
- Oyster sauce can be bought in the Asian section of most supermarkets.

countdown

- Marinate veal.
- Boil rice.
- Prepare all the stir-fry ingredients.
- Stir-fry veal dish.
- Finish mange tout and rice.

stir-fried veal

Artificial sweetener equivalent to 2 teaspoons sugar
2 tablespoons oyster sauce
2 medium garlic cloves, crushed
350g (12oz) veal escalopes, cut into 2.5cm (1in) pieces
1 teaspoon cornflour
2 teaspoons sesame oil
1/2 medium cucumber, peeled and cut into 2.5cm (1in) pieces
1 medium grapefruit, cut into segments
2 tablespoons unsweetened grapefruit juice from fresh grapefruit
Salt and freshly ground black pepper

Mix the sweetener, oyster sauce and garlic together. Marinate the veal in the mixture for 10 minutes. Sprinkle cornflour over veal and toss. The marinade will be absorbed by the veal. Heat sesame oil in a wok or frying pan. Make sure wok is very hot. Add veal and stir-fry for 2 minutes. Remove from wok and add cucumber, grapefruit and grapefruit juice. Boil to thicken sauce for 1 minute. Return veal to wok and remove from heat. Add salt and pepper to taste. Serve over mange tout and rice.
Makes 2 servings.

Per serving: 483 calories, 46.4 grams protein, 19.3 grams carbohydrate, 22.9 grams fat (11.6 saturated), 150 milligrams cholesterol, 370 milligrams sodium, 1.8 grams fibre

mange tout and rice

50g (2oz) 30-minute quick-
cooking brown rice

110g (4oz) mange tout, trimmed

1 teaspoon sesame oil

Salt and freshly ground black
pepper

Fill a large saucepan with about 2–3 litres
(4–5 pints) water. Add rice and bring to the boil.
Boil for 20 minutes then add the mange tout.
Continue to boil for 2–3 minutes. Drain. Toss
with sesame oil and salt and pepper to taste.
Serve with the veal.

Makes 2 servings.

Per serving: 132 calories, 4.3 grams protein,
22.3 grams carbohydrate, 3.2 grams fat
(0.5 saturated), 0 milligrams cholesterol, 3 milligrams
sodium, 2.6 grams fibre

shopping list

FRUIT AND VEG

110g (4oz) mange tout

1 medium cucumber

1 medium grapefruit

MEAT

350g (12oz) veal escalopes

GROCERY

1 small bottle oyster sauce

1 small bottle sesame oil

STAPLES

30-minute quick-cooking
brown rice

Garlic

Artificial sweetener

Cornflour

Salt

Black peppercorns

five-spice tuna tataki

Tataki – beef or fish that has been seared, thinly sliced, chilled and served with a dipping sauce – is a tangy, Japanese recipe. Traditional tataki accompaniments are grated daikon (white radish), ginger, chopped spring onions and a dipping sauce.

Japanese and Chinese rice vinegars are made from fermented rice. They're milder than most Western vinegars. White vinegar can be used in this recipe. Add a few drops of water to soften the strength.

Brown rice takes about 45 minutes to cook. There are several brands of quick-cooking brown rice available. Their cooking time ranges from 10 to 30 minutes. I find the 30-minute rice has more flavour, but any quick-cooking rice will work for this dinner.

helpful hints

- *Coarse-ground black pepper and five-spice powder can be bought in the spice section of the supermarket.*
- *Red radishes can be used instead of the daikon or white radish.*

countdown

- *Sear tuna and let cool slightly.*
- *Make rice.*
- *While rice cooks, prepare sauce.*
- *Make dessert just before serving.*

five-spice tuna tataki

2 x 175g (6oz) tuna steaks
1 tablespoon coarse-ground black pepper
1¹/₂ tablespoons sesame oil
2 tablespoons low-sodium soy sauce
2 medium garlic cloves, crushed
¹/₂ teaspoon five-spice powder
1 small daikon (white) radish, grated (optional)

Roll tuna steaks in black pepper. Heat _ tablespoon sesame oil in a small non-stick frying pan over high heat. Sear tuna for 2 minutes. Turn and sear second side for 2 minutes. Remove to a chopping board and thinly slice.

Mix soy sauce, remaining tablespoon sesame oil, garlic and five-spice powder together in a small bowl. Serve sliced tuna on 2 individual dinner plates and spoon sauce on top. Sprinkle with grated daikon radish.
Makes 2 servings.

Per serving: 335 calories, 37.3 grams protein,
2.5 grams carbohydrate, 18.0 grams fat
(3.4 saturated), 59 milligrams cholesterol,
677 milligrams sodium, 0 grams fibre

japanese brown rice

50g (2oz) 30-minute quick-
   cooking brown rice
110g (4oz) button mushrooms,
   sliced
110g (4oz) fresh mange tout,
   trimmed
115ml (4fl oz) fat-free, low-sodium
   chicken stock
1 tablespoon rice vinegar
2 tablespoons low-sodium soy
   sauce
Salt and freshly ground black
   pepper

Bring a large saucepan with 2–3 litres (4–5 pints)
of water to the boil. Add rice and boil for 25
minutes. Add mushrooms and mange tout and
continue to boil for 5 minutes. Drain. Mix
chicken stock, vinegar and soy sauce together
and toss with rice and vegetables. Add salt and
pepper to taste.
Makes 2 servings.

Per serving: 125 calories, 6.1 grams protein,
22.1 grams carbohydrate, 1.1 grams fat
(0.1 saturated), 0 milligrams cholesterol,
750 milligrams sodium, 2.4 grams fibre

raspberry banana cooler

110g (4oz) frozen raspberries
   (not in sugar syrup)
1/2 medium banana, sliced
225ml (8fl oz) diet lemon-lime
225ml (8fl oz) ice cubes
Artificial sweetener equivalent to
   2 teaspoons sugar

Place raspberries, banana, diet lemon-lime, ice
cubes and sweetener in a blender or food
processor and blend until smooth. Serve in tall
glasses.
Makes 2 servings.

Per serving: 66 calories, 1.1 grams protein,
16.4 grams carbohydrate, 0.6 grams fat
(0.1 saturated), 0 milligrams cholesterol,
1 milligram sodium, 3.5 grams fibre

shopping list

FRUIT AND VEG
   1 small daikon (white) radish
   1 medium banana
   110g (4oz) button
      mushrooms
   110g (4oz) fresh mange tout
SEAFOOD
   2 x 175g/6oz tuna steaks
GROCERY
   1 small jar five-spice powder
   1 small pack frozen
      raspberries (not in sugar
      syrup)
   1 small can/bottle diet
      lemon-lime
   1 small bottle rice vinegar
   1 small jar coarse-ground
      black pepper
   1 small bottle sesame oil
STAPLES
   Garlic
   Quick-cooking brown rice
   Artificial sweetener
   Fat-free, low-sodium chicken
      stock
   Low-sodium soy sauce
   Salt
   Black peppercorns

helpful hints

- *Look for roasted chicken that is not marinated in honey or a barbecue sauce. These sauces usually contain sugar.*
- *This recipe calls for serving the chicken at room temperature. For a hot meal, microwave chicken on high for 2 minutes.*

countdown

- *Start rice.*
- *Make salsa.*
- *Assemble salad.*

chicken with black bean salsa and brown rice

Roasted chicken served over rice with a black bean and corn salsa dresses up shop-bought roasted or rotisserie chicken breasts.

Sweet vermouth gives this black bean and corn salsa an intriguing flavour. Use the salsa dressing in the recipe or add vermouth and cumin to a bottled low-fat vinaigrette dressing. Brown rice takes about 45 minutes to cook. There are several brands of quick-cooking brown rice available. Their cooking time ranges from 10 to 30 minutes. I find the 30-minute rice has more flavour, but any quick-cooking rice will work for this dinner.

brown rice

4oz (110g) 30-minute quick-
cooking brown rice
1 tablespoon plus 1 teaspoon
rapeseed oil,
1/2 tablespoon plus 1 teaspoon
sweet (rosso) vermouth
Salt and freshly ground black
pepper

First, prepare the brown rice. Bring a large saucepan with 2–3 litres (4–5 pints) of water to the boil. Add rice and boil, uncovered, for about 30 minutes (or follow packet instructions). Drain into a sieve in the sink. Run hot water through rice and stir with a fork. Return rice to saucepan and add 1 teaspoon rapeseed oil, 1 teaspoon vermouth and salt and pepper to taste.

chicken with black bean salsa

1 teaspoon ground cumin

Several drops hot pepper sauce

50g (2oz) tinned black beans, rinsed and drained

50g (2oz) frozen corn kernels, defrosted

350g (12oz) roasted chicken breast, bones and skin removed

15g (1/2oz) chopped fresh coriander

2 small tomatoes, cut into wedges

Salt and freshly ground black pepper

While rice cooks, mix 1 tablespoon rapeseed oil, tablespoon vermouth, cumin, hot pepper sauce and salt and pepper to taste in a medium-sized bowl. Add the black beans and corn. Toss well. Taste and add more seasoning if needed. Spoon rice on to 2 dinner plates. Slice chicken and place on rice. Spoon salsa on top and sprinkle with coriander. Arrange tomatoes on the side of the dinner plates.

Makes 2 servings.

Per serving: 558 calories, 32.0 grams protein, 38.4 grams carbohydrate, 18.4 grams fat (3.2 saturated), 144 milligrams cholesterol, 146 milligrams sodium, 2.6 grams fibre

shopping list

FRUIT AND VEG

   1 small bunch coriander

   2 small tomatoes

MEAT

   350g (12oz) roasted chicken breast, bones and skin removed

GROCERY

   1 small bottle sweet (rosso) vermouth

   1 small tin black beans

   1 small pack frozen corn kernels

STAPLES

   Quick-cooking brown rice

   Rapeseed oil

   Ground cumin

   Hot pepper sauce

   Salt

   Black peppercorns

veal piccata

Tender veal escalopes are sautéed in a wine and lemon sauce for this quick meal. Garlic courgettes and tomatoes take only minutes in the microwave oven.

helpful hints

- The vegetables can be sautéed instead of cooking them in a microwave oven. Heat the oil in a non-stick frying pan, add the vegetables, cover with a lid, and cook for 10 minutes.

countdown

- Boil water for orzo.
- Prepare all ingredients.
- Boil orzo.
- While orzo boils, microwave vegetables.
- Sauté veal.

veal piccata

2 tablespoons flour
Salt and freshly ground black
    pepper
350g (12oz) veal escalopes
1 teaspoon olive oil
2 tablespoons fresh lemon juice
2 tablespoons dry vermouth
50ml (2fl oz) fat-free, low-sodium
    chicken stock
2 tablespoons chopped fresh
    parsley (optional)

Season flour with salt and pepper to taste. Dip veal in flour and shake off excess. Heat oil in a medium-sized non-stick frying pan on medium-high heat. When oil is very hot, brown veal on both sides, about 1 minute per side. Sprinkle lemon juice on top. Remove veal to a plate and cover with foil to keep warm. Raise heat to high and add vermouth and chicken stock to the pan. Reduce the liquid by half, takes about 3 minutes. Add salt and pepper to taste. Spoon sauce over veal and sprinkle with parsley.
Makes 2 servings.

Per serving: 424 calories, 44.2 grams protein, 12.4 grams carbohydrate, 19.1 grams fat (10.4 saturated),138 milligrams cholesterol, 177 milligrams sodium, 0.6 grams fibre

garlic courgettes and tomato orzo

50g (2oz) orzo (rice-shaped pasta)

225g (8oz) courgettes, cut into
2.5cm (1in) pieces

1 medium tomato, cut into 2.5cm
(1in) pieces

2 medium garlic cloves, crushed

2 teaspoons olive oil

Salt and freshly ground black
pepper

Bring a large saucepan filled with 3–4 litres (5–7 pints) water to the boil. Add orzo and boil for 8 minutes. Drain. Meanwhile, place courgettes, tomatoes and garlic in a microwave-safe bowl. Cover with clingfilm or a plate and microwave on high for 3 minutes. Remove, stir and microwave on high for 1 minute. Remove and add orzo, olive oil and salt and pepper to taste. Toss well.

Makes 2 servings.

Per serving: 157 calories, 4.5 grams protein,
23.3 grams carbohydrate, 5.1 grams fat
(0.7 saturated), 0 milligrams cholesterol,
6 milligrams sodium, 1.2 grams fibre

shopping list

FRUIT AND VEG

1 small bunch parsley
(optional)

225g (8oz) courgettes

1 medium tomato

MEAT

350g (12oz) veal escalopes

GROCERY

1 small bottle dry vermouth

1 small pack orzo

STAPLES

Lemons

Garlic

Flour

Olive oil

Fat-free, low-sodium chicken
stock

Salt

Black peppercorns

right carbs

Great food that's great for you is the goal of this third phase, which is designed to become your permanent lifestyle. This is an overall balanced approach to eating. The right-carb phase approximates to a 40-30-30 dietary profile. While there are differences of opinion, it is generally agreed that fat levels (primarily mono-unsaturated) should make up to 30 per cent of one's diet. Carbohydrate intake should be restricted to 30 per cent more than protein intake. So if the calories from protein are 30 per cent of one's diet, the correct carbohydrate level should be 40%. Here in these recipes, high-fibre carbohydrates are incorporated into breakfast, lunch and dinner menus.

Following the Right Carb 14-Day Meal Plan you will consume an average of 135-145 grams of carbohydrates per day. Carbohydrate percentage is based on carbohydrates less fibre consumed, which is the normal way of calculating carbohydrate consumption. The balance of these meals is 39 per cent of calories from carbohydrates, 31 per cent of calories from lean protein, 20 per cent of calories from mono-unsaturated fat and 6 per cent of calories from unsaturated fat.

As with the other sections, I have organised the menus into a meal-at-a-glance chart with some easy and quick meals for mid-week and those that take a little more time for the weekends. They are arranged to give variety throughout the day and over the course of the week. Presentation is as ever important and the appeal of a beautiful plate of food adds to our eating experience. Celebrating events and holidays with friends and cooking for them is a pleasure and almost all the recipes here can be used for special occasions.

Breakfast

Mediterranean Scramble on Toast and Monte Cristo Sandwich are two of the savoury breakfasts you can choose from. Try them all to add variety to your morning repertoire. Your body does need a boost of energy in the morning to set you up for the day, both mentally and physically, so don't skimp here.

Lunch

Choose from the wide variety to fit every appetite. When you're in a hurry, grab a BLT Sandwich on Rye or Chicory and Orange Salad with Swiss Turkey. The quality of the ingredients is important with simply prepared food. When you have more time, enjoy the Blue Cheese and Beef Pasta Salad.

Dinner

Enjoy these meals without worrying about numbers or questioning what you eat. The old saying that you should breakfast like a King, lunch like a Prince and dine like a Pauper is one of the best pieces of nutritional advice ever given. Menus like Whisky-Soused Salmon and Turkey Gratinée will entice you to stay on this low-carbohydrate, balanced style of eating. Roasted Pepper and Olive Snapper makes a delicious and rounded meal good enough for a King!

For those days when you are really pressed for time, select Mock Hungarian Goulash or Black Bean Soup with Rice from the Super Speed Suppers section of the book. For weekends when you have more time and want something special, try the Pan-Seared Tuna with Mango Salsa, or Indian-Spiced Chicken from the Weekends section of the book.

right carbs 14-day meal plan at a glance

week 1	breakfast	lunch	dinner
sunday	Ham and Pepper Frittata 95	Mulligatawny Soup 103	Pan-Seared Tuna with Mango Salsa..............158
monday	Smoked Salmon Sandwich...................96	BLT Sandwich on Rye.............................104	Chicken Creole..........136
tuesday	Strawberry Splash with Cottage Cheese-Stuffed Chicory 97	Layered Antipasto Salad 105	Mahi Mahi Satay with Thai Peanut Sauce.............112
wednesday	Microwave Portobello Scramble 98	Blue Cheese and Beef Pasta Salad...........................106	Turkey-Gratinée with Basil Linguine...................114
thursday	Mediterranean Scramble on Toast 99	Chicory and Orange Salad with Swiss Turkey 107	Parmesan Sole...........135
friday	Monte Cristo Sandwich 100	Mushroom and Sausage Soup..........................108	Roast Pork with Strawberry Salsa..........................111
saturday	Provençal Omelette 101	Danish Prawn Smorrebrod 109	Indian-Spiced Chicken....................157

week 2	breakfast	lunch	dinner
sunday	Ham and Pepper Frittata 95	Mulligatawny Soup 103	Whisky-Soused Salmon 116
monday	Smoked Salmon Sandwich....................96	BLT Sandwich on Rye............................104	Roasted Pepper and Olive Snapper 118
tuesday	Strawberry Splash with Cottage Cheese-Stuffed Chicory 97	Layered Antipasto Salad 105	Hawaiian Chicken with Pineapple Caesar Salad.........................120
wednesday	Microwave Portobello Scramble 98	Blue Cheese and Beef Pasta Salad.........................106	Black Bean Soup with Rice............................138
thursday	Mediterranean Scramble on Toast 99	Chicory and Orange Salad with Swiss Turkey 107	Mock Hungarian Goulash....................139
friday	Monte Cristo Sandwich 100	Mushroom and Sausage Soup...........................108	Mexican Sopes 122
saturday	Provençal Omelette 101	Danish Prawn Smorrebrod 109	Pork Chops with Apple Relish......................160

right carbs
breakfasts

ham and pepper frittata

Plump, juicy frittatas take about 10 minutes to make. They can be made ahead and eaten at room temperature. They differ from omelettes. An omelette is cooked quickly over high heat, making it creamy and runny, while a frittata is cooked slowly over low heat, making it firm and set. A frittata needs to be cooked on both sides. It can be flipped over in the pan, but a much easier way is to place it in the oven or under a grill for half a minute to finish cooking.

ham and pepper frittata

Olive oil spray
225g (8oz) sliced onion
175g (6oz) sliced lean ham, cut into bite-sized pieces
1 medium red pepper, sliced
225ml (8fl oz) egg substitute
Salt and freshly ground black pepper

Pre-heat grill. Heat an ovenproof medium-sized non-stick frying pan on medium-high heat and spray with olive oil spray. Add onion, ham and red pepper. Cook for 2 minutes. Mix egg substitute with salt and pepper to taste. Reduce heat to low and add egg mixture. Cook, without browning the bottom, for 10 minutes. The eggs will be set, but the top a little runny. Place pan under the grill for $1/2$–1 minute until the top is set, but not brown. Remove and cut in half. Slide halves on to 2 plates.
Makes 2 servings.

bran cereal

225ml (8fl oz) skimmed milk
75g (3oz) high-fibre, no-sugar-added bran cereal

Divide ingredients between 2 cereal bowls.
Makes 2 servings.

vegetable juice

350ml (12fl oz) low-sodium, no-sugar-added tomato or V-8 juice

Divide between 2 glasses.
Makes 2 servings.

Per serving: 366 calories, 38.1 grams protein, 50.6 grams carbohydrate, 7.6 grams fat (2.3 saturated), 42 milligrams cholesterol, 1178 milligrams sodium, 14.5 grams fibre

helpful hints

● *Be careful when removing the frying pan from the grill. The handle will be very hot and remain hot for several minutes after it is removed. Place a pot holder or oven glove over the handle for safety.*

countdown

● *Pre-heat the grill.*
● *Make frittata.*
● *While frittata cooks, assemble cereal.*

shopping list

FRUIT AND VEG
   1 medium red pepper
DELI
   175g (6oz) sliced lean ham
STAPLES
   Onion
   Egg substitute
   Olive oil spray
   Skimmed milk
   High-fibre, no-sugar-added bran cereal
   Low-sodium, no-sugar-added tomato or V-8 juice
   Salt
   Black peppercorns

helpful hints

- *Smoked salmon can be frozen. Scottish, Norwegian or Atlantic salmon can be used.*

countdown

- *Make oatmeal.*
- *Assemble smoked salmon sandwich.*

shopping list

FRUIT AND VEG
   1 medium tomato
DAIRY
   1 small carton reduced-fat
      cream cheese
SEAFOOD
   175g (6oz) smoked salmon
STAPLES:
   Rye bread
   Skimmed milk
   Oatmeal
   Artificial sweetener

smoked salmon sandwich

Buttery, smooth smoked salmon is a special breakfast treat.

smoked salmon sandwich

2 slices rye bread
2 tablespoons reduced-fat cream
   cheese
175g (6oz) smoked salmon
1 medium tomato, sliced

Toast rye bread and spread with cream cheese. Divide smoked salmon in half and place over cream cheese on each piece of toast. Serve sandwiches with sliced tomato on the side. *Makes 2 servings.*

oatmeal

75g (3oz) oatmeal
450ml (16fl oz) water
225ml (8fl oz) skimmed milk
Artificial sweetener equivalent to
   2 teaspoons sugar (optional)

To prepare in the microwave, combine oatmeal and water together. Microwave on high for 4 minutes. Stir in milk and sweetener. Alternatively, combine oatmeal and water in a small saucepan. Bring to the boil. Cook for about 5 minutes over medium heat, stirring occasionally. Stir in milk and sweetener. *Makes 2 servings.*

Per serving: 416 calories, 28.7 grams protein, 50.7 grams carbohydrate, 11.0 grams fat (4.9 saturated), 39 milligrams cholesterol, 985 milligrams sodium, 5.6 grams fibre

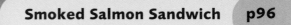

Smoked Salmon Sandwich   **p96**

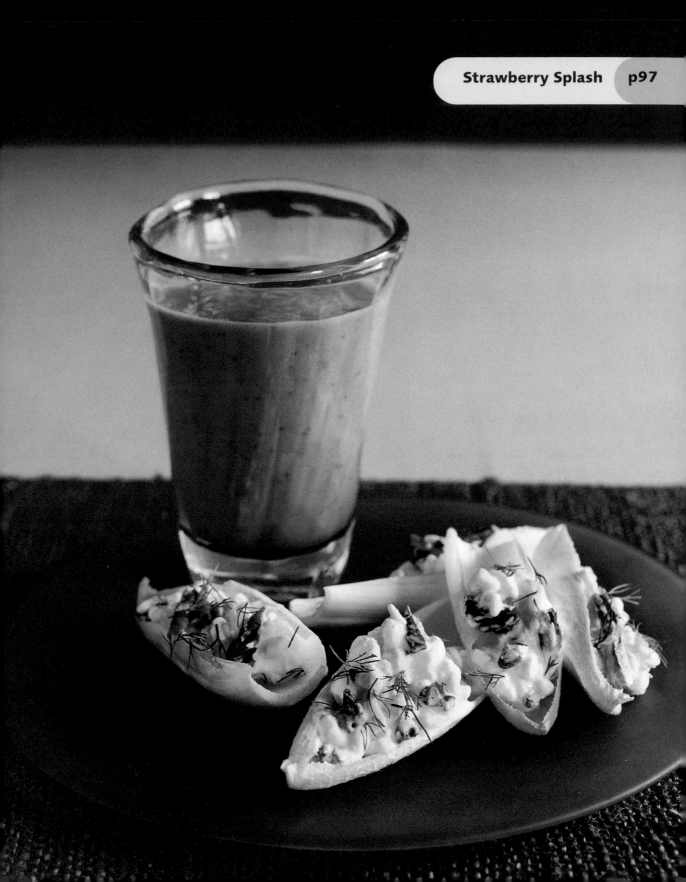

Strawberry Splash p97

strawberry splash

Sweet strawberries flavour this quick shake that you can make and take on the run.

strawberry splash

225ml (8fl oz) soya milk
275g (10oz) strawberries
1 teaspoon vanilla essence
Artificial sweetener equivalent to
 2 teaspoons sugar

Place soya milk, strawberries, vanilla essence and sweetener in a blender and blend until smooth. Divide between 2 glasses.
Makes 2 servings.

cottage cheese-stuffed chicory

225g (8oz) low-fat cottage cheese
2 tablespoons pecan pieces
2 tablespoons snipped dill or
 ¹/₂ teaspoon dried
1 small head chicory

Mix cottage cheese, pecans and dill together. Remove leaves from chicory and fill with cottage cheese mixture. Divide between 2 plates.
Makes 2 servings.

bran cereal

225ml (8fl oz) skimmed milk
75g (3oz) high-fibre, no-sugar-
 added bran cereal

Divide ingredients between 2 cereal bowls.
Makes 2 servings.

Per serving: 387 calories, 24.6 grams protein, 54.8 grams carbohydrate,13.7 grams fat (2.6 saturated), 12 milligrams cholesterol, 610 milligrams sodium, 16.9 grams fibre

helpful hints

- *Frozen or fresh strawberries can be used. Make sure frozen ones are not packed in sugar syrup.*
- *Use any type of berries.*
- *The stuffed chicory can be made the night before and wrapped in clingfilm.*
- *The easiest way to chop dill leaves is to snip them right off the stem with scissors.*
- *Dried dill can be used.*

countdown

- *Make shake.*
- *Assemble stuffed chicory.*

shopping list

FRUIT AND VEG
 1 punnet strawberries
  (275g/10oz needed)
 1 small bunch fresh dill (or
  dried dill in a jar)
 1 small head chicory
DAIRY
 1 small carton soya milk
  (225ml/8fl oz needed)
 225g (8oz) low-fat cottage
  cheese
GROCERY
 1 small bottle vanilla essence
 1 small packet pecan pieces
STAPLES
 Skimmed milk
 Artificial sweetener
 High-fibre, no-sugar-added
  bran cereal

microwave portobello scramble

The earthy flavour of the portobello mushrooms and the distinctive taste of Parmesan cheese give these microwaved scrambled eggs a rich flavour.

microwave portobello scramble

2 slices rye bread
110g (4oz) sliced portobello mushrooms
2 teaspoons olive oil
225ml (8fl oz) egg substitute
3 tablespoons Parmesan cheese
Pinch grated nutmeg
Salt and freshly ground black pepper

Toast rye bread and place on 2 plates. Place mushrooms in a microwave-safe bowl and drizzle with olive oil. Microwave on high for 1 minute. Whisk together egg substitute, Parmesan cheese, nutmeg and salt and pepper to taste in a bowl. Remove mushrooms from microwave and stir. Pour in egg mixture and stir. Return bowl to microwave oven and microwave on high for 1½ minutes. Remove and stir. Return for another 1 minute. Divide into two portions and spoon on to toast.
Makes 2 servings.

bran cereal

225ml (8fl oz) skimmed milk
75g (3oz) high-fibre, no-sugar-added bran cereal

Divide ingredients between 2 cereal bowls.
Makes 2 servings.

Per serving: 365 calories, 27.3 grams protein, 49.1 grams carbohydrate, 11.5 grams fat (3.7 saturated), 13 milligrams cholesterol, 894 milligrams sodium, 14.9 grams fibre

mediterranean scramble on toast

Seasoned olives chopped and mixed with spices provide a savoury accent for these quick scrambled eggs on toast.

mediterranean scramble on toast

2 slices wholemeal bread
2 tablespoons olive tapenade
Olive oil spray
225ml (8fl oz) egg substitute
2 tablespoons grated Parmesan
   cheese
Freshly ground black pepper

Toast bread and spread with olive tapenade. Heat a small non-stick frying pan on medium-high heat and spray with olive oil spray. Mix egg substitute with Parmesan cheese and pepper to taste. Pour into pan and cook for 2–3 minutes or until eggs are set. Divide in half and spoon on toast.
Makes 2 servings.

oatmeal

75g (3oz) oatmeal
450ml (16fl oz) water
225ml (8fl oz) skimmed milk
Artificial sweetener equivalent to
   2 teaspoons sugar (optional)

To prepare in the microwave, combine oatmeal and water together. Microwave on high for 4 minutes. Stir in milk and sweetener. Alternatively, combine oatmeal and water in a small saucepan. Bring to the boil. Cook about 5 minutes over medium heat, stirring occasionally. Stir in milk and sweetener.
Makes 2 servings.

Per serving: 383 calories, 29.2 grams protein, 46.3 grams carbohydrate, 9.4 grams fat (2.8 saturated), 9 milligrams cholesterol, 700 milligrams sodium, 7 grams fibre

helpful hints

● *Buy good-quality Parmesan cheese and grate it yourself or chop it in the food processor. Freeze extra for quick use. You can quickly spoon out what you need and leave the rest frozen.*

countdown

● *Toast bread and spread with olive tapenade.*
● *Make eggs.*

shopping list

GROCERY
   1 small jar olive tapenade
STAPLES
   Egg substitute
   Parmesan cheese
   Skimmed milk
   Oatmeal
   Olive oil spray
   Wholemeal bread
   Artificial sweetener
   Black peppercorns

monte cristo sandwich

Here's a quick version of an old American staple made with cheese and turkey, dipped in batter and fried or baked.

monte cristo sandwich

2 slices reduced-fat Swiss or Gruyère cheese (50g /2oz)
2 slices turkey breast (25g/1oz)
4 slices wholemeal bread
225ml (8fl oz) egg substitute
Salt and freshly ground black pepper to taste
Olive oil spray

Place 1 slice Swiss cheese and 1 slice turkey on 1 slice of bread. Cover with second slice of bread. Repeat with remaining cheese, turkey and bread. Beat egg substitute with salt and pepper to taste. Dip closed sandwiches into egg mixture. Place a large non-stick frying pan over medium heat and spray with olive oil spray. Remove sandwiches from egg mixture and place in frying pan. Brown for 2 minutes and turn. Cover with a lid and cook for2 minutes more. Remove to 2 plates, cut sandwiches in half, and serve.
Makes 2 servings.

bran cereal

225ml (8fl oz) skimmed milk
75g (3oz) high-fibre, no-sugar-added bran cereal

Divide ingredients between 2 cereal bowls.
Makes 2 servings.

Per serving: 372 calories, 40.2 grams protein, 52.5 grams carbohydrate, 8.9 grams fat (3.1 saturated), 27 milligrams cholesterol, 707 milligrams sodium, 19 grams fibre

helpful hints

● *Buy turkey breast without added sugar. Honey-coated and barbecued turkey should be avoided as the glazes are sugar based.*

countdown

● *Make sandwich.*
● *Assemble cereal.*

shopping list

DAIRY
   1 small packet reduced-fat Swiss or Gruyère cheese (50g/2oz needed)
DELI
   1 small packet sliced turkey breast
STAPLES
   Egg substitute
   Olive oil spray
   Wholemeal bread
   High-fibre, no-sugar-added bran cereal
   Skimmed milk
   Salt
   Black peppercorns

provençal omelette

The flavours of this omelette remind me of sunny Provence where thyme, parsley, peppers and tomatoes grow abundantly in the rich soil.

provençal omelette

2 slices multi-grain bread
Olive oil spray
1/2 teaspoon dried thyme
50g (2oz) chopped fresh parsley
115ml (4 fl oz) low-sodium, no-sugar-added tomato sauce
2 whole eggs
4 egg whites
1/8 teaspoon cayenne pepper
Salt and freshly ground black pepper

Toast bread, spray with olive oil spray, and set aside. Mix thyme, parsley and tomato sauce together and set aside. Heat a medium-sized non-stick frying pan over medium-high heat. Place eggs in a bowl and stir in cayenne pepper and salt and pepper to taste. Pour the mixture into the frying pan. Let the eggs set for about 30 seconds. Tip the pan and lightly move the eggs so that they all set. Cook for 1½ minutes or until eggs are set. Cook a few seconds longer for firmer eggs. Spoon tomato sauce on half the omelette and fold the omelette in half. Slide out of the pan by tipping the pan and holding a plate vertically against the side of the pan. Turn the pan and plate to invert the omelette on to the plate. Cut in half and serve on 2 plates with the toast.
Makes 2 servings.

oatmeal

75g (3oz) oatmeal
450ml (16fl oz) water
225ml (8fl oz) skimmed milk
Artificial sweetener equivalent to 2 teaspoons sugar (optional)

To prepare in the microwave, combine oatmeal and water together. Microwave on high for 4 minutes. Stir in milk and sweetener. Alternatively, combine oatmeal and water in a small saucepan. Bring to the boil. Cook about 5 minutes over medium heat, stirring occasionally. Stir in milk and sweetener.
Makes 2 servings.

Per serving: 380 calories, 28.9 grams protein, 50.1 grams carbohydrate, 11.2 grams fat (2.6 saturated), 215 milligrams cholesterol, 373 milligrams sodium, 7.8 grams fibre

helpful hints

● *Dried thyme is called for. If using dried spices, make sure the bottle is less than 6 months old.*

countdown

● *Make oatmeal.*
● *Make omelette.*

shopping list

FRUIT AND VEG
  110g (4oz) portobello mushrooms
  1 medium tomato
DELI
  110g (4oz) smoked turkey breast
STAPLES
  Eggs (6 needed)
  Olive oil spray
  Dried tarragon
  Salt
  Black peppercorns

right carbs
lunches

mulligatawny soup

Curry powder and ginger give mulligatawny soup a pungent flavour, while chicken and freshly diced crunchy apple provide a contrast in textures.

Authentic curry powder is a blend of freshly ground spices and herbs such as cardamom, chillies, cinnamon, cloves, coriander and cumin and is made fresh every day. Commercial curry powder comes in two forms: standard and Madras, the hotter one.

This soup tastes great the second day. If you have time, make double the recipe and reheat when you want to use it.

mulligatawny soup

2 teaspoons rapeseed oil
225g (8oz) sliced onion
1 medium carrot, sliced
1 celery stalk, sliced
$\frac{1}{2}$ tablespoon curry powder
1 tablespoon flour
1cm ($\frac{1}{2}$in) piece fresh ginger, chopped or 1 teaspoon ground ginger
350ml (12fl oz) fat-free, low-sodium chicken stock
225ml (8fl oz) water
115ml (4fl oz) 'light' coconut milk
225g (8oz) roasted boneless, skinless chicken breast pieces
Salt and freshly ground black pepper
1 medium apple, cored and cubed
2 tablespoons chopped fresh coriander (optional)
4 lemon wedges

Heat oil on medium-high heat in a large non-stick saucepan. Add onion, carrot and celery. Sauté for 5 minutes. Add the curry powder, flour and ginger and sauté for about 30 seconds. Stir in chicken stock, water and coconut milk and simmer for 5 minutes. Add chicken and continue to simmer for another 5 minutes. Add salt and pepper to taste. Spoon into 2 bowls. Sprinkle with chopped apple and coriander. Place lemon wedges on side.

Makes 2 servings.

Per serving: 337 calories, 32.5 grams protein, 28.8 grams carbohydrate, 12.5 grams fat (3.5 saturated), 72 milligrams cholesterol, 547 milligrams sodium, 2.7 grams fibre

dessert

2 medium pears

Divide between 2 dessert plates.

Makes 2 servings.

Per serving: 98 calories, 0.7 grams protein, 25.1 grams carbohydrate, 0.7 grams fat (0 saturated), 0 milligrams cholesterol, 1 milligram sodium, 4.1 grams fibre

helpful hints

● Curry powder can be found in the spice section of the supermarket. It loses its freshness after 2–3 months.
● The soup tastes even better after letting it stand. Leave it for about 5–10 minutes and reheat if you have time.

countdown

● Make soup.
● Assemble dessert.

shopping list

FRUIT AND VEG
1 medium apple
1 small bunch fresh coriander (optional)
1 small piece fresh ginger (or ground ginger)
2 medium pears
MEAT
225g (8oz) roasted boneless, skinless chicken breast pieces
GROCERY
1 small jar curry powder
1 tin 'light' coconut milk (115ml/4fl oz needed)
STAPLES
Carrot
Celery
Lemon
Onion
Rapeseed oil
Flour
Fat-free, low-sodium chicken stock
Salt
Black peppercorns

BLT sandwich on rye

This bacon, rocket and tomato on rye bread is a modern version of the classic American bacon, lettuce and tomato sandwich.

BLT sandwich on rye

225g (8oz) back bacon, cut into 5cm (2in) strips

2 slices rye bread

2 tablespoons reduced-fat mayonnaise

1 tablespoon frozen chopped onion, defrosted

75g (3oz) fresh rocket, torn into bite-sized pieces

1 medium tomato, sliced

Heat a medium-sized non-stick frying pan on medium-high heat and add bacon strips. Sauté for 2–3 minutes. Remove to a plate. Meanwhile, toast bread and mix mayonnaise with onion. Spread toast with mayonnaise mixture. Divide rocket into 2 servings and place on toast. Place tomato slices on the rocket. Top with bacon strips. Serve as open sandwiches.
Makes 2 servings.

Per serving: 305 calories, 26.6 grams protein, 22.5 grams carbohydrate, 11.9 grams fat (3.2 saturated), 58 milligrams cholesterol, 1321 milligrams sodium, 1.9 grams fibre

dessert

550g (1¼lb) watermelon cubes

Divide between 2 dessert bowls.
Makes 2 servings.

Per serving: 99 calories, 1.9 grams protein, 22.1 grams carbohydrate, 1.3 grams fat (0.2 saturated), 0 milligrams cholesterol, 6 milligrams sodium, 1.5 grams fibre

helpful hints

- *Any type of salad leaves can be used instead of rocket.*
- *Bacon can be cooked in microwave for 1 minute.*
- *Frozen onion can be defrosted in the microwave for 2 minutes.*
- *Fresh-cut watermelon cubes can be found in the fruit and veg section of some supermarkets.*

countdown

- *Sauté bacon.*
- *Toast bread.*
- *Assemble sandwich.*

shopping list

FRUIT AND VEG

1 container fresh watermelon cubes

1 bunch rocket

1 medium tomato

DELI

225g (8oz) back bacon

STAPLES

Rye bread

Reduced-fat mayonnaise

Frozen chopped onion

layered antipasto salad

Prawns, Parmesan curls, tomatoes, roasted red pepper, rocket and lettuce form colourful layers for this antipasto salad that is topped with a flavourful Italian dressing.

layered antipasto salad

2 medium tomatoes

2 tablespoons no-sugar-added oil
  and vinegar dressing

275g (10oz) washed, ready-to-eat
  Italian-style salad leaves

2 medium green peppers, cut into
  rings

450g (16oz) sweet pepper,
  drained and cut into strips

40g (1¹/₂oz) rocket, torn into large
  pieces

2 tablespoons Parmesan curls

225g (8oz) peeled, deveined and
  cooked prawns

225g (8oz) red onion rings

Quarter 1 tomato and place in food processor with oil and vinegar dressing. Process to make a sauce. Place salad leaves in a salad bowl. Cover with a layer of sliced green pepper. Spread the sweet pepper on top of the green pepper and layer the rocket on top. Slice the second tomato and place it over the rocket. Make Parmesan curls by scraping a potato peeler over the cheese. Place prawns and Parmesan curls over rocket. Sprinkle with onion rings and dressing mixture. *Makes 2 servings.*

> Per serving: 387 calories, 33.3 grams protein,
> 31.8 grams carbohydrate, 13.5 grams fat
> (3.5 saturated), 181 milligrams cholesterol,
> 466 milligrams sodium, 0.4 grams fibre

dessert

1 grapefruit

Cut grapefruit in half with a serrated knife and cut around edge and between segments. Place each half on a dessert plate and serve. *Makes 2 servings.*

> Per serving: 39 calories, 0.8 grams protein, 9.9 grams
> carbohydrate, 0.1 gram fat (0 saturated), 0 milligrams
> cholesterol, 0 milligrams sodium, 1.3 grams fibre

helpful hints

- *Get cooked, peeled prawns from the fish counter or frozen food section. Make sure they are of good quality.*
- *Look for washed, ready-to-eat salad selections with many different-coloured leaves.*
- *Any type of bowl can be used for the salad. A glass one shows off the coloured layers.*
- *Make Parmesan strips by peeling thin strips from the cheese with a potato peeler.*

countdown

- *Prepare ingredients.*
- *Make salad.*

shopping list

FRUIT AND VEG
  2 medium tomatoes
  1 bag washed, ready-to-eat
    Italian-style salad leaves
  2 medium green peppers
  1 small bunch rocket
  1 grapefruit
SEAFOOD
  225g (8oz) peeled, deveined
    and cooked prawns
GROCERY
  1 jar sweet peppers
STAPLES
  Parmesan cheese
  No-sugar-added oil and
    vinegar dressing
  Red onion

helpful hints

- Any short-cut pasta can be used.
- Ask the deli counter to slice the roast beef in one thick slice. It is easier to cut into cubes this way.

countdown

- Boil water.
- While pasta cooks, prepare remaining ingredients.

shopping list

FRUIT AND VEG
  1 medium pear
  1 small bunch grapes
  1 packet cherry tomatoes
DAIRY
  1 packet blue cheese
DELI
  110g (4oz) roast beef
GROCERY
  1 small packet wholemeal penne pasta or other short-cut pasta (75g/3oz needed)
STAPLES
  No-sugar-added oil and vinegar dressing
  Salt
  Black peppercorns

blue cheese and beef pasta salad

Pasta tossed with sweet ripe pears, tangy blue cheese and juicy roast beef makes this colourful and tasty lunch.

blue cheese and beef pasta salad

75g (3oz) wholemeal penne pasta
1 medium pear, cored and sliced into 2.5cm (1in) pieces
110g (4oz) cubed roast beef
250g (9oz) cherry tomatoes
2 tablespoons no-sugar-added oil and vinegar dressing
Salt and freshly ground black pepper
3 tablespoons crumbled blue cheese

Bring a large saucepan filled with water to the boil. Add the pasta and cook for 10 minutes, or according to packet instructions. Do not overcook. Drain into a colander in the sink and run under cold water. Place in a bowl and add pear slices, roast beef and tomatoes. Add dressing and salt and pepper to taste. Toss well. Sprinkle blue cheese on top.
Makes 2 servings.

Per serving: 393 calories, 25.0 grams protein, 37.0 grams carbohydrate, 17.4 grams fat (5.6 saturated), 57 milligrams cholesterol, 318 milligrams sodium, 5.6 grams fibre

dessert

1 small bunch grapes

Divide the grapes between 2 dessert bowls.
Makes 2 servings.

Per serving: 58 calories, 0.6 grams protein, 15.8 grams carbohydrate, 0.3 grams fat (0.1 saturated), 0 milligrams cholesterol, 2 milligrams sodium, 0 grams fibre

chicory and orange salad with swiss turkey

Chicory and orange segments make a colourful and quick salad. To make this ahead, assemble the salad and the Swiss Turkey, but add the dressing and melt the cheese on the sandwiches just before serving.

chicory and orange salad

2 medium heads chicory
2 medium oranges
1 tablespoon pinenuts
2 tablespoons olive oil and vinegar dressing

Wipe chicory with damp kitchen paper. Cut 2.5cm (1in) from the base end of the chicory. Slice the chicory crossways and place in a bowl. Peel oranges and break or cut into segments. Add to bowl. Place pinenuts on a small foil-lined baking tray and toast under grill. Sprinkle over salad. Drizzle with dressing. Divide between 2 plates. *Makes 2 servings.*

Per serving: 165 calories, 1.7 grams protein, 18.3 grams carbohydrate, 8.9 grams fat (2.2 saturated), 0 milligrams cholesterol, 93 milligrams sodium, 3.2 grams fibre

swiss turkey

110g (4oz) sliced turkey breast
2 slices multi-grain bread
25g (1oz) sliced reduced-fat Swiss or Gruyère cheese
1 medium tomato, sliced

Place turkey on bread and place sliced cheese on top. Place on foil-lined baking tray under a grill for 2 minutes or until cheese melts. Divide between 2 plates and place tomato slices on the side. Serve with chicory salad. *Makes 2 servings.*

Per serving: 193 calories, 26 grams protein, 12.8 grams carbohydrate, 5.1 grams fat (1.9 saturated), 48 milligrams cholesterol, 181 milligrams sodium, 3 grams fibre

melon cup

425g (15oz) melon cubes

Divide melon cubes between 2 dessert bowls. *Makes 2 servings.*

Per serving: 86 calories, 2.1 grams protein, 20.1 grams carbohydrate, 0.6 grams fat (0 saturated), 0 milligrams cholesterol, 21 milligrams sodium, 0.8 grams fibre

helpful hints

- *Any type of salad leaf can be used instead of the chicory.*
- *Cubed fresh melon can be found in the fruit and veg section of most supermarkets.*

countdown

- *Pre-heat grill.*
- *Make salad.*
- *Spoon melon into dessert bowls.*
- *Make sandwich.*

shopping list

FRUIT AND VEG
  2 medium heads chicory
  1 tomato
  2 medium oranges
  425g (15oz) melon cubes
DAIRY
  1 small packet sliced reduced-fat Swiss or Gruyère cheese (25g/1oz needed)
DELI
  110g (4oz) sliced turkey breast
GROCERY
  1 small packet pinenuts
  Multi-grain bread
STAPLES
  Olive oil and vinegar dressing

helpful hints
- *Any type of mushrooms can be used.*

countdown
- *Make soup.*
- *While soup cooks, assemble dessert.*

shopping list
FRUIT AND VEG
   450g (1lb) portobello
      mushrooms
   4 clementines
MEAT
   225g (8oz) low-fat turkey
      sausages
STAPLES
   Olive oil
   Onion
   Fat-free, low-sodium chicken
      stock
   Grated nutmeg
   Salt
   Black peppercorns

mushroom and sausage soup

Mushrooms and sweet sausages make this a warm and hearty lunch. Make extra and use the next day or freeze.

mushroom and sausage soup

2 teaspoons olive oil
450g (1lb) sliced onion
225g (8oz) low-fat turkey
   sausages, cut into 2.5cm (1in)
   pieces
450g (1lb) portobello mushrooms,
   sliced
350ml (12fl oz) fat-free, low-
   sodium chicken stock
1/2 teaspoon grated nutmeg
Salt and freshly ground black
   pepper

Heat oil in a large saucepan on medium-high heat. Add onion and sausage. Sauté for 5 minutes. The onions will be transparent, not brown. Add the mushrooms and sauté for 3 minutes. Add the chicken stock and bring to a simmer. Cook for 15 minutes. Add nutmeg and salt and pepper to taste. Taste and add more nutmeg, if needed.
Makes 2 servings.

> Per serving: 349 calories, 25.0 grams protein, 20.2 grams carbohydrate, 16.1 grams fat (3.4 saturated), 60 milligrams cholesterol, 1146 milligrams sodium, 2.5 grams fibre

dessert

4 clementines

Divide between 2 plates and serve.
Makes 2 servings.

> Per serving: 74 calories, 1 gram protein, 18.8 grams carbohydrate, 0.4 grams fat (0 saturated), 0 milligrams cholesterol, 2 milligrams sodium, 3.9 grams fibre

danish prawn smorrebrod

Pretty Danish open sandwiches are attractive and good to eat too.

danish prawn smorrebrod

1 tablespoon mayonnaise

1 tablespoon freshly squeezed
   lemon juice

225g (8oz) peeled, deveined and
   cooked prawns, sliced

Salt and freshly ground black
   pepper

2 slices rye bread

2 red-leaf lettuce leaves

150g (5oz) diced tomato

Mix mayonnaise and lemon juice together. Add prawns and salt and pepper to taste. Toss well. Place rye bread on 2 plates. Place a lettuce leaf on each slice. Spoon prawns on top. Sprinkle diced tomatoes on prawns.

Makes 2 servings.

Per serving: 263 calories, 26.5 grams protein, 18.8 grams carbohydrate, 8.6 grams fat (1.4 saturated), 176 milligrams cholesterol, 423 milligrams sodium, 1.9 grams fibre

scandinavian cucumber salad

Artificial sweetener equivalent to
   1 teaspoon sugar

6 tablespoons hot water

2 tablespoons distilled white
   vinegar

2 tablespoons fresh dill, chopped,
   or 1 teaspoon dried

1 teaspoon freshly ground black
   pepper

1 medium cucumber, peeled and
   thinly sliced

Dissolve the artificial sweetener in hot water. When thoroughly dissolved, add vinegar, dill and black pepper. Mix well. Pour over cucumber and leave to marinate for 10 minutes. Serve with sandwich.

Makes 2 servings.

Per serving: 26 calories, 0.9 grams protein, 6.1 grams carbohydrate, 0.3 grams fat (0 saturated), 0 milligrams cholesterol, 4 milligrams sodium, 0.9 grams fibre

blueberry cup

350g (12oz) blueberries

Divide blueberries between 2 dessert bowls.

Makes 2 servings.

Per serving: 82 calories, 1 gram protein, 20 grams carbohydrate, 0.5 grams fat (0 saturated), 0 milligrams cholesterol, 9 milligrams sodium, 4.4 grams fibre

helpful hints

- The quickest way to chop fresh dill is to snip the leaves from the stem with scissors.
- Any type of leaf lettuce can be used.
- Slice cucumber in a food processor fitted with a thin slicing blade. Or thinly slice with a mandoline.

countdown

- Make cucumber salad and leave to marinate while preparing sandwich.
- Make sandwich.

shopping list

FRUIT AND VEG
   1 medium cucumber
   1 medium tomato
   1 small head red-leaf lettuce
   1 small bunch fresh dill (or
      dried dill)
   1 small punnet blueberries

SEAFOOD
   225g (8oz) peeled, deveined
      and cooked prawns

STAPLES
   Lemon
   Rye bread
   Mayonnaise
   Artificial sweetener
   Distilled white vinegar
   Salt
   Black peppercorns

right carbs
dinners

roast pork with strawberry salsa

Pork fillet with chunky strawberry salsa makes a sweet and spicy dinner. Strawberries, normally used for dessert, can also be added to salads or used to make tasty condiments for cooked meats.

roast pork with strawberry salsa

350g (12oz) pork fillet

Olive oil spray

1½ teaspoons ground cumin

275g (10oz) ripe strawberries, hulled and cut into 0.5cm (¼in) pieces

Artificial sweetener equivalent to 1 teaspoon sugar

50g (2oz) diced red onion

Several drops hot pepper sauce

1 tablespoon fresh lime juice

Salt

4 tablespoons chopped fresh coriander (optional)

Pre-heat grill. Line a baking tray with foil and place under grill. Trim fat from pork and cut filet in half lengthways. Spray all sides with olive oil spray. Sprinkle with 1 teaspoon ground cumin. Remove baking tray from grill and place pork on tray. Grill for 5 minutes. Turn and cook for another 5 minutes. Test pork. A meat thermometer should read 70ºC/160ºF. While pork grills, place strawberries in a medium-sized bowl and sprinkle with sweetener. Add onion and hot pepper sauce. Mix the remaining ½ teaspoon cumin and lime juice together and drizzle over berries. Add salt to taste. Toss well and sprinkle with coriander. Serve pork with salsa on top.
Makes 2 servings.

> Per serving: 333 calories, 46.7 grams protein, 13.8 grams carbohydrate, 10.1 grams fat (3.3 saturated), 146 milligrams cholesterol, 115 milligrams sodium, 2.8 grams fibre

courgettes and linguine

110g (4oz) spinach linguine

225g (8oz) courgettes, halved lengthways and sliced

225g (8oz) diced red onion

1 tablespoon olive oil

Salt and freshly ground black pepper

Place a large saucepan filled with 3–4 litres (5–7 pints) of water on to boil. Add the pasta and boil for 5 minutes. Add the courgettes and onion and continue to boil for 3 minutes, or until the pasta is cooked through but firm. Drain the pasta and vegetables leaving a few tablespoons of cooking water with the pasta. Toss with the olive oil. Add salt and pepper to taste.
Makes 2 servings.

> Per serving: 316 calories, 9.4 grams protein, 52.3 grams carbohydrate, 7.9 grams fat (1.1 saturated), 0 milligrams cholesterol, 6 milligrams sodium, 3.5 grams fibre

helpful hints

- *If you like your salsa hot, add more pepper sauce.*
- *Any type of berry can be used.*
- *Placing the pork on a pre-heated baking tray helps it to cook faster.*
- *Red onion is used in both recipes. Dice at one time and divide accordingly.*
- *If you come across them, use yellow courgettes instead of green, to add a contrasting colour to the dish.*

countdown

- *Pre-heat grill and baking tray.*
- *Boil water for pasta.*
- *Grill pork.*
- *Make salsa.*
- *Boil pasta and courgettes.*

shopping list

FRUIT AND VEG

1 small punnet ripe strawberries (275g/10oz needed)

1 lime

1 small bunch fresh coriander (optional)

225g (8oz) courgettes

MEAT

350g (12oz) pork fillet

GROCERY

110g (4oz) spinach linguine

STAPLES

Olive oil spray

Olive oil

Ground cumin

Artificial sweetener

Red onions

Hot pepper sauce

Salt

Black peppercorns

helpful hints

● *Any firm fish such as monkfish, swordfish or cod can be used.*

● *Rice vinegar can be bought in the Asian section of the supermarket. Half a tablespoon water mixed with tablespoon distilled white vinegar may be used as a substitute.*

● *An easy way to marinate the fish is to place the marinade and fish in a self-closing plastic bag. You can easily turn the bag halfway through the marinade time to make sure all of the fish is marinated.*

countdown

● *Pre-heat grill.*
● *Marinate fish.*
● *Start rice.*
● *Make sauce for fish.*
● *Grill fish.*
● *Finish rice dish.*

mahi mahi satay with thai peanut sauce

Fresh fish, quickly cooked and served with a spicy, peanut sauce, brings back memories of the enticing aroma of satay (Asian kebabs) cooking on small grills in the street markets of South-east Asia. I've used peanut butter as a base for the spicy peanut sauce to shorten the preparation time.

If using wooden skewers, be sure to soak them in water for about 30 minutes before use. This keeps them from burning under the grill.

The fish only takes 4 minutes to cook.

Brown rice takes about 45 minutes to cook. There are several brands of quick-cooking brown rice available. Their cooking time ranges from 10 to 30 minutes. I find the 30-minute rice has more flavour, but any quick-cooking rice will work for this dinner.

mahi mahi satay with thai peanut sauce

1 teaspoon rapeseed oil
1 tablespoon rice vinegar
1½ garlic cloves, bruised
Salt and freshly ground black
  pepper
350g (12oz) mahi mahi
2 x 20cm (8in) wooden or metal
  skewers
2 tablespoons crunchy peanut
  butter
1 tablespoon low-sodium soy
  sauce
Artificial sweetener equivalent to
  2 teaspoons sugar
6 drops hot pepper sauce

Pre-heat grill. Mix oil, 1 tablespoon rice vinegar and garlic together. Add salt and pepper to taste. Slice fish into strips about 1cm (½ in) thick and 10cm (4in) long. Place in the marinade and set aside for 10 minutes, turning after 5 minutes to make sure all sides are marinated. Remove from marinade and thread the fish strips on to the skewers. I find that threading in a wave pattern allows more even cooking. Place on a foil-lined baking tray and grill for 2 minutes on each side.

To make the peanut sauce: In a small bowl, mix peanut butter, soy sauce and remaining _ tablespoon rice vinegar together until blended to a smooth consistency. Add artificial sweetener and hot pepper sauce.

Serve the skewers on a plate with a little of the sauce poured over the fish and the rest on the side for dipping.

Makes 2 servings.

Per serving: 259 calories, 33.8 grams protein,
4.6 grams carbohydrate, 11.6 grams fat
 (2.1 saturated), 116 milligrams cholesterol,
446 milligrams sodium, 0 grams fibre

mange tout and rice

*50g (2oz) 30-minute quick-
   cooking brown rice*
110g (4oz) mange tout, trimmed
2 teaspoons rapeseed oil
*Salt and freshly ground black
   pepper*

Bring a large saucepan filled with 2–3 litres (4–5 pints) of water to the boil. Add the rice, stir once or twice, and let boil for 25 minutes. Add the mange tout and continue to boil for 2 minutes. Test a grain; rice should be cooked through, but not soft. Drain into a sieve in the sink and return to the pan. Mix in oil and salt and pepper to taste.
Makes 2 servings.

Per serving: 153 calories, 4.3 grams protein, 22.3 grams carbohydrate, 5.5 grams fat (0.8 saturated), 0 milligrams cholesterol, 3 milligrams sodium, 2.6 grams fibre

lychee cup

*350g (12oz) tinned, drained
   lychees*

Divide between 2 dessert bowls.
Makes 2 servings.

Per serving: 126 calories, 2 grams protein, 32 grams carbohydrate, 0.5 grams fat (0 saturated), 0 milligrams cholesterol, 2 milligrams sodium, 4 grams fibre

shopping list
FRUIT AND VEG
   110g (4oz) mange tout
SEAFOOD
   350g (12oz) mahi mahi
GROCERY
   1 small bottle rice vinegar
   *1 small jar crunchy peanut
      butter*
   *1 small packet 20cm (8in)
      wooden or metal skewers*
   1 tin lychees
STAPLES
   Rapeseed oil
   Garlic
   *30-minute quick-cooking
      brown rice*
   Low-sodium soy sauce
   Artificial sweetener
   Hot pepper sauce
   Salt
   Black peppercorns

turkey gratinée with basil linguine

A golden, cheesy crust tops this quick turkey and mushroom sauté. The grilled grated cheese and breadcrumb crust is called a gratin. This meal takes about 10 minutes to complete. Or you can make it ahead and then place it under the grill just before you need it.

The turkey breast escalopes called for in the recipe are cut about 0.5cm (1/4in) thick. They only need to be cooked for 1 minute on each side. Watch them carefully. They become dry and tough if overdone.

helpful hints

- Buy good-quality Parmesan cheese and grate it yourself or chop it in the food processor. Freeze extra for quick use. You can quickly spoon out what you need and leave the rest frozen.
- Chicken escalopes can be substituted for turkey.
- Any green herb can be substituted for the basil.
- Fresh pineapple cubes can be found in the fruit and veg section of many supermarkets.

countdown

- Pre-heat grill.
- Make dessert.
- Boil water for pasta.
- Make turkey.
- Make pasta.

turkey gratinée

1 teaspoon olive oil
225g (8oz) turkey breast escalopes (about 0.5cm/1/4 inch thick)
Salt and freshly ground black pepper
225g (8oz) frozen chopped onion
2 medium garlic cloves, crushed
225g (8oz) portobello mushrooms, sliced
1 tablespoon flour
115ml (4fl oz) skimmed milk
25g (1oz) plain breadcrumbs
2 tablespoons grated Parmesan cheese

Pre-heat grill. Heat oil in a medium-sized non-stick ovenproof frying pan over medium-high heat. Brown turkey for 1 minute, then turn and brown second side for 1 minute. Remove to a plate and sprinkle with salt and pepper to taste. Add onion, garlic and mushrooms to pan and sauté for 2 minutes. Add flour and continue to sauté for 30 seconds. Add milk and stir for 2 minutes to thicken sauce. Push mushrooms to sides of frying pan and return turkey to the pan. Cover turkey with mushrooms and sprinkle with breadcrumbs and Parmesan cheese. Add salt and pepper to taste. Place under grill for 2 minutes.
Makes 2 servings.

Per serving: 355 calories, 41.3 grams protein, 18.7 grams carbohydrate, 10.2 grams fat (3.5 saturated), 88 milligrams cholesterol, 312 milligrams sodium, 0 grams fibre

basil linguine

110g (4oz) fresh linguine
2 teaspoons olive oil
15g (1oz) chopped fresh basil
Salt and freshly ground black
*   pepper*

Bring a large saucepan filled with 3–4.5 litres (6–8 quarts) of water to the boil. When water comes to the boil, add pasta and cook 3 minutes for fresh pasta or 9 minutes for dried. Drain, leaving about 2 tablespoons pasta water with the pasta. Add olive oil to pasta and toss well. Add basil and salt and pepper to taste.
Makes 2 servings.

Per serving: 219 calories, 5.8 grams protein, 35.7 grams carbohydrate, 5.4 grams fat (0.7 saturated), 0 milligrams cholesterol, 1 milligram sodium, 2.1 grams fibre

spiced pineapple

teaspoon ground allspice
Artificial sweetener equivalent to
*   2 teaspoons sugar*
275g (10oz) pineapple cubes

Mix allspice and sweetener together. Place pineapple cubes in a microwave-safe bowl. Sprinkle spice mixture on top and toss to make sure all cubes are coated with the mixture. Place in microwave oven and microwave on high for 1 minute. Remove and divide between 2 dessert bowls.
Makes 2 servings.

Per serving: 77 calories, 0.6 grams protein, 20.2 grams carbohydrate, 0.7 grams fat (0 saturated), 0 milligrams cholesterol, 1 milligrams sodium, 2.4 grams fibre

shopping list

FRUIT AND VEG
   1 small bunch fresh basil
   225g (8oz) sliced portobello
   *   mushrooms*
   1 container pineapple cubes
MEAT
   225g (8oz) turkey breast
   *   escalopes (about*
   *   0.5cm/¼in thick)*
GROCERY
   1 small jar ground allspice
   110g (4oz) fresh linguine
   1 small packet plain
   *   breadcrumbs*
STAPLES
   Olive oil
   Garlic
   Frozen chopped onions
   Skimmed milk
   Flour
   Parmesan cheese
   Artificial sweetener
   Salt
   Black peppercorns

whisky-soused salmon

Salmon, potatoes and whisky combine to star in this quick dinner. Salmon can be bought as thick steaks with the bone in or as thin fillets.

helpful hints

- *The quickest way to wash watercress is to place it leaves first into a bowl of water. Leave for a minute, then lift out and shake dry.*
- *A quick way to chop chives is to cut them with scissors.*

countdown

- *Make dessert*
- *Boil potatoes.*
- *Make salmon sauce.*
- *Poach salmon.*
- *Add broccoli and finish potatoes.*

whisky-soused salmon

2 x 175g (6oz) salmon steaks
450ml (16fl oz) water
Pinch salt
50ml (2 fl oz) reduced-fat mayonnaise
1 tablespoon fresh lemon juice
1 tablespoon whisky
Several sprigs of watercress

Rinse salmon. Bring water to the boil and add salt. Place salmon in water. Liquid should completely cover salmon. Add more water, if needed. Bring to a simmer and gently cook for 5 minutes. Salmon will be opaque. Remove to individual plates. Whisk mayonnaise, lemon juice and whisky together in a small bowl and spoon over salmon. Place several sprigs of watercress on the side.
Makes 2 servings.

Per serving: 286 calories, 38.6 grams protein, 0.8 grams carbohydrate, 9.8 grams fat (2.3 saturated), 111 milligrams cholesterol, 114 milligrams sodium, 0 grams fibre

broccoli and potatoes

225g (8oz) new potatoes, washed and cut into 3.5cm (1¹/₂in) pieces
110g (4oz) broccoli florets
2 teaspoons olive oil
Salt and freshly ground black pepper
2 tablespoons snipped chives

Place potatoes in a large saucepan and cover with cold water. Cover with a lid and bring to the boil. Lower heat to medium and simmer for 5 minutes. Add the broccoli florets and continue to cook, covered, for 5 minutes. Drain, remove to a bowl, and toss with olive oil and salt and pepper to taste. Sprinkle with chives. Toss well. *Makes 2 servings.*

Per serving: 159 calories, 5.1 grams protein, 25.2 grams carbohydrate, 5.1 grams fat (0.6 saturated), 0 milligrams cholesterol, 27 milligrams sodium, 3.0 grams fibre

deep dish blueberry cream

1 tablespoon cornflour
Artificial sweetener equivalent to 2 teaspoons sugar
350g (12oz) blueberries
225ml (8fl oz) water
225ml (8fl oz) non-fat vanilla yoghurt

In a small cup, mix cornflour and sugar. Stir this mixture into water placed in a medium-sized saucepan. Bring to the boil over high heat and allow to thicken. Add 50g (2oz) blueberries and boil for 3 minutes. Remove from heat. Divide yoghurt between 2 ramekins. Spoon the remaining berries on top. Spoon sauce over berries. Refrigerate until needed. *Makes 2 servings.*

Per serving: 192 calories, 6.5 grams protein, 41.6 grams carbohydrate, 0.6 grams fat (0 saturated), 3 milligrams cholesterol, 104 milligrams sodium, 4.4 grams fibre

shopping list

FRUIT AND VEG
225g (8oz) new potatoes
1 small packet broccoli florets
1 small bunch fresh chives
1 small bunch watercress
1 small punnet blueberries
DAIRY
1 pot non-fat vanilla yoghurt
SEAFOOD
2 x 175g (6oz) salmon steaks
GROCERY
1 small bottle whisky
STAPLES
Olive oil
Reduced-fat mayonnaise
Lemon
Cornflour
Artificial sweetener
Salt
Black peppercorns

roasted pepper and olive snapper

Fresh snapper, roasted red peppers and Greek olives are grilled for only 8 minutes for this simple Greek meal. This quick meal was inspired by a trip to Greece. We drove to Delphi along a road bordered by an endless sea of olive trees. These amazing groves contained over a million trees. The view over this olive carpet leading to the blue sea was spectacular. Brown rice takes about 45 minutes to cook. There are several brands of quick-cooking brown rice available. Their cooking time ranges from 10 to 30 minutes. I find the 30-minute rice has more flavour, but any quick-cooking rice will work for this dinner.

roasted pepper and olive snapper

2 x 175g (6oz) snapper fillets
1 tablespoon olive oil
Salt and freshly ground black pepper
350g (12oz) sliced sweet pepper, drained
8 stoned black olives, cut in half

Pre-heat grill. Wash fish fillets and pat dry with kitchen paper. Place in a small, shallow ovenproof dish. Drizzle olive oil on top. Sprinkle with salt and pepper to taste. Place pimiento slices and olives around fish. Grill for 8 minutes. If fillet is 2.5cm (1in) thick, grill for 10 minutes. Serve fish on 2 plates and spoon roasted peppers and olives on top.
Makes 2 servings.

Per serving: 296 calories, 33.6 grams protein, 15.2 grams carbohydrate, 11.5 grams fat (1.5 saturated), 57 milligrams cholesterol, 694 milligrams sodium, 3 grams fibre

lemon-braised celery hearts and rice

225ml (8fl oz) fat-free, low-sodium chicken stock

225ml (8fl oz) water

6 medium celery stalks, tender lower sections only, cut into 5cm (2in) pieces

50g (2oz) 30-minute quick-cooking brown rice

1 tablespoon freshly squeezed lemon juice

2 teaspoons olive oil

40g (1½oz) raisins

Salt and freshly ground black pepper

Pour chicken stock and water into a saucepan and bring to the boil on high heat. Add celery and rice and reduce heat to medium. Cover with a lid and simmer for 30 minutes until stalks are tender but still firm. Drain, reserving 3 tablespoons liquid. Remove to a shallow bowl. Mix lemon juice, olive oil and cooking liquid together and add raisins, salt and pepper to taste. Pour over rice and celery.

Makes 2 servings.

Per serving: 184 calories, 3.4 grams protein, 33.1 grams carbohydrate, 5.5 grams fat (0.8 saturated), 0 milligrams cholesterol, 54 milligrams sodium, 1 gram fibre

peach crumble

3 medium peaches, stones removed and sliced

2 tablespoons flour

Artificial sweetener equivalent to 2 teaspoons sugar

1 tablespoon butter

Place peach slices in an oven-to-table bowl that can also be used in a microwave oven. Microwave fruit on high for 2 minutes. Mix flour and sweetener together. Cut in butter, and rub with fingertips to make a crumbly mixture. Spoon over fruit and place under grill for 5 minutes, or until topping is golden.

Makes 2 servings.

Per serving: 138 calories, 1.8 grams protein, 21.6 grams carbohydrate, 5.7 grams fat (3.5 saturated), 16 milligrams cholesterol, 58 milligrams sodium, 0.8 grams fibre

shopping list

FRUIT AND VEG
  1 bunch celery hearts
  3 medium peaches
SEAFOOD
  2 x 175g (6oz) snapper fillets
GROCERY
  1 jar sweet peppers
  1 container stoned black
    olives (8 olives needed)
  1 small packet raisins
STAPLES
  Olive oil
  Butter
  Flour
  30-minute quick-cooking
    brown rice
  Fat-free, low-sodium chicken
    stock
  Artificial sweetener
  Lemon
  Salt
  Black peppercorns

hawaiian chicken with pineapple caesar salad

On a trip to Hawaii I met a famous local chef who served me a Hawaiian chicken dish with a pineapple barbecue glaze. I've adapted his ideas for these recipes. Barbecue sauces can be filled with sugar. Here's one you can make with a sweet flavour and not many carbs.
Brown rice takes about 45 minutes to cook. There are several brands of quick-cooking brown rice available. Their cooking time ranges from 10 to 30 minutes. I find the 30-minute rice has more flavour, but any quick-cooking rice will work for this dinner.

helpful hints

- *Fresh pineapple cubes can be found in the fruit and veg section of many supermarkets.*
- *Look for no-sugar-added pineapple juice.*
- *I have cooked this chicken in a frying pan, because it's faster and easier than heating the grill for a mid-week dinner. If you have the time, grill the chicken for about 2 minutes per side then move it to a cooler area of the grill. Add a spoonful of sauce to each piece and cook for 2 more minutes.*
- *To cube a mango, slice off each side as close to the stone as possible. Take the mango half in your hand, skin side down. Score the fruit in a criss-cross pattern through to the skin. Bend the skin backwards so that the cubes pop up. Slice the cubes away from the skin. Repeat with the other half. Score and slice any fruit left on the stone.*

countdown

- *Make dessert and set aside.*
- *Make chicken sauce.*
- *Cook chicken.*
- *Make salad.*

hawaiian chicken

2 x 175g (6oz) boneless, skinless chicken breasts
Olive oil spray
Salt and freshly ground black pepper
50ml (2fl oz) no-sugar-added pasta sauce
2 tablespoons pineapple juice
2 teaspoons Dijon mustard
Artificial sweetener equivalent to 2 teaspoons sugar
75g (3oz) 30-minute quick-cooking brown rice
1 teaspoon rapeseed oil

Place chicken between 2 layers of greaseproof paper and flatten with a kitchen mallet or the bottom of a heavy pan. Heat a medium-sized non-stick frying pan on medium-high heat and spray with olive oil spray. Brown chicken for 2 minutes. Turn and brown for another 2 minutes. Season both sides with salt and pepper. Lower heat to medium and spoon 1 tablespoon sauce over each piece. Cover with a lid and cook for 2 minutes. A meat thermometer should read 80ºC/170ºF. Remove to 2 dinner plates and serve remaining sauce on the side.
Makes 2 servings.

Per serving: 379 calories, 52.4 grams protein, 19.8 grams carbohydrate, 10.5 grams fat (2.1 saturated), 132 milligrams cholesterol, 336 milligrams sodium, 1.3 grams fibre

pineapple caesar salad

275g (10oz) pineapple cubes

150g (5oz) romaine lettuce, torn into bite-sized pieces

15g (¹/₂oz) snipped chives

2 tablespoons no-sugar-added Caesar dressing

2 tablespoons grated Parmesan cheese

Place pineapple cubes and lettuce in a salad bowl. Add chives and dressing. Toss well. Sprinkle the top with Parmesan cheese. *Makes 2 servings.*

Per serving: 162 calories, 1.5 grams protein, 20.6 grams carbohydrate, 9.7 grams fat (1.5 saturated), 18 milligrams cholesterol, 124 milligrams sodium, 2.6 grams fibre

dessert

2 medium mangoes cut into cubes

Divide mangoes between 2 dessert bowls. *Makes 2 servings.*

Per serving: 134 calories, 1.1 grams protein, 35.2 grams carbohydrate, 0.6 grams fat (0.1 saturated), 0 milligrams cholesterol, 4 milligrams sodium, 2.2 grams fibre

shopping list

FRUIT AND VEG
- 1 container fresh pineapple cubes (275g/10oz needed)
- 1 small head romaine lettuce
- 1 small bunch chives
- 2 medium mangoes

MEAT
- 2 x 175g (6oz) boneless, skinless chicken breasts

GROCERY
- 1 small jar/tin pineapple juice
- 1 bottle no-sugar-added Caesar dressing

STAPLES
- Parmesan cheese
- Olive oil spray
- Rapeseed oil
- No-sugar-added pasta sauce
- Dijon mustard
- 30-minute quick-cooking brown rice
- Artificial sweetener
- Salt
- Black peppercorns

mexican sopes

On a trip to Mexico City, I watched a local chef make these melt-in-your-mouth sopes. They're little corn tortillas filled with a spicy black bean spread, roasted chicken, lettuce and cheese. Although sopes are usually served as appetisers, she mentioned that they make quick and easy supper dishes too.

mexican sopes

helpful hints

- *Any type of salsa can be used. Choose the heat of the salsa according to your preference.*
- *Buy washed, ready-to-eat, shredded lettuce.*
- *If all 4 tortillas don't fit into your frying pan, cook them in batches.*
- *If pressed for time, use a bought jar of spicy black bean dip instead of making the spread in the recipe.*

countdown

- *Make Oranges in Cherry Coulis and set aside.*
- *Make black bean spread.*
- *Shred chicken and prepare ingredients.*
- *Make sopes.*

2 teaspoons rapeseed oil
110g (4oz) diced red onion
110g (4oz) rinsed and drained tinned black beans
Several drops hot pepper sauce
Salt and freshly ground black pepper
225g (8oz) roasted or rotisserie chicken breast, skin and bones removed
4 x 15cm (6in) corn tortillas
75g (3oz) washed, ready-to-eat, shredded lettuce
25g (1oz) grated reduced-fat Cheddar cheese
225ml (8fl oz) medium-heat no-sugar-added tomato salsa

Heat 1 teaspoon oil in a large non-stick frying pan on medium-high heat. Add half the diced onion and sauté until it starts to shrivel, about 3 minutes. Remove to the bowl of a food processor. Add beans, remaining 1 teaspoon oil and hot pepper sauce and purée. If you do not have a food processor, mash the beans with a fork and mix with the onion, oil and hot pepper sauce. If the beans are dry, add a few tablespoons of water. Add salt and pepper to taste. Set aside. Shred chicken into bite-sized pieces.

Place the same frying pan over medium-low heat. Add the tortillas and warm for 30 seconds. Turn them over and spread the top of each tortilla with the black bean mixture. Sprinkle with the remaining onion. Layer lettuce, cheese and chicken over each one. If tortillas do not all fit in pan, cook them 2 at a time. Cover with a lid for 1 minute. Remove to 2 dinner plates. Spoon salsa on top or serve on the side.
Makes 2 servings.

Per serving: 517 calories, 54.8 grams protein, 49.8 grams carbohydrate, 15.6 grams fat (4.1 saturated), 104 milligrams cholesterol, 1112 milligrams sodium, 8.0 grams fibre

oranges in cherry coulis

2 oranges
*275g (10oz) frozen sweet, dark
    cherries*

Peel oranges and slice over a bowl to catch the juice. Defrost cherries for 1 minute in a microwave oven. Purée cherries in a food processor, adding juice from peeled oranges, or press cherries through a food mill. Spoon cherry coulis on to 2 dessert plates. Place orange slices on top.
Makes 2 servings.

Per serving: 228 calories, 31.5 grams protein, 4.7 grams carbohydrate, 9.3 grams fat (2.5 saturated), 253 milligrams cholesterol, 215 milligrams sodium, 0 grams fibre

shopping list

FRUIT AND VEG
    *1 bag washed, ready-to-eat
        shredded lettuce*
    2 oranges
DAIRY
    *1 packet grated reduced-fat
        Cheddar cheese*
MEAT
    *225g (8oz) roasted or
        rotisserie chicken breast*
GROCERY
    *1 bag frozen sweet, dark
        cherries*
    4 x 15cm (6in) corn tortillas
STAPLES
    Rapeseed oil
    Red onion
    Tinned black beans
    Hot pepper sauce
    *Medium-heat, no-sugar-
        added tomato salsa*
    Salt
    Black peppercorns

super speed suppers

These meals are for those nights when I haven't got the time to think about dinner, but don't want to send out for something that won't fit my low-carb lifestyle. At the end of the day, when I've just come in and the family needs to be fed, I need a repertoire of super speed suppers that can just be thrown together. It's a good idea to keep a stock of items that are the base of many super speed dishes – like fresh lettuce, from cos to romaine, and radicchio and rocket to add varied colour and flavour. I've based the recipes in this section on ingredients that I bought from the supermarket that can be assembled into a meal in 15 minutes or less.

Savoury Sage Chicken is one of my real favourites and I have made it time and again over the years since first moving to a low-carb lifestyle. It's based on roasted or rotisserie chicken that is tarted up at home and you'd be surprised just how much zing it has from the addition of a little dry vermouth. It fits the Quick Start nutritional guidelines and takes about 10 minutes to make from start to finish. Delicious!

I love a good, hearty bowl of soup for supper, even in the summer. The Peasant Country Soup is perfect for a quick dinner. It takes only 10 minutes to make and fits the Which Carb nutritional guidelines. Full of robust flavours, it is deeply satisfying.

When I brought the Mock Hungarian Goulash to the radio station studio for one of my programmes, all the staff lined up for seconds. It is made in 10 minutes, uses lean roast beef from the deli, and fits the Right Carbs nutritional guidelines.

Simply prepared food can be just as satisfying as something that's taken hours to make. Shopping is important and choosing the best ingredients you can afford will enhance the pleasure of eating good fresh dishes.

Look for ingredients which have not been covered in sauces and seasonings to cover up for poor quality. Look for vegetables and fruits in season and ring the changes – one of the Super Speed Lunch menus includes melon for dessert and, if you look at the array of different melons in the supermarket, you will see that it is easy to choose a new variety for each day of the week.

These meals have been incorporated into the 2-week menu plan for the appropriate phase. Keep a good store of bottled ingredients on hand and you can throw a dinner together faster than getting into your car or phoning for a take-away. Jerk seasoning, tomato salsa, teriyaki sauce and Worcestershire sauce are just some of those to have around all the time; there is no end of low-carb ideas that can be made speedily using them.

When I give cooking classes and show these ideas, the response is always surprising – that you can get such flavourful food in such a short time. I've served these meals at dinner parties, too, without telling anyone they were low-carb.

quick start

super speed

suppers

greek prawns with feta cheese

This meal fits the nutritional guidelines for the Quick Start phase. Greek feta cheese gives this prawn dish a tangy Mediterranean flavour.

greek prawns with feta cheese

2 teaspoons olive oil

110g (4oz) frozen chopped onion

2 garlic cloves, crushed

1 large tomato, diced

350g (12oz) large prawns, shelled
    and deveined

50g (2oz) crumbled feta cheese

1 teaspoon dried oregano

Salt and freshly ground black
    pepper

Heat olive oil in a medium-sized non-stick frying pan on medium-high heat and add the onion, garlic and tomato. Sauté for 3 minutes. Add prawns and sprinkle cheese and oregano on top. Sauté for 3 minutes, turning prawns to make sure they are cooked on both sides. Remove from heat, cover with a lid, and let sit for 2 minutes, or until cheese melts. Add salt and pepper to taste.

Makes 2 servings.

> Per serving: 349 calories, 41.6 grams protein, 9.6 grams carbohydrate, 14.9 grams fat (6.2 saturated), 280 milligrams cholesterol, 638 milligrams sodium, 0.9 grams fibre

cos and fresh cabbage salad

175g (6oz) shredded, washed,
    ready-to-eat cabbage

175g (6oz) shredded, washed,
    ready-to-eat cos lettuce

2 spring onions, sliced

1 teaspoon dried dill

2 tablespoons olive oil and vinegar
    dressing

Combine cabbage, lettuce, spring onions and dill in a bowl. Add dressing and toss well.

Makes 2 servings.

> Per serving: 104 calories, 1.4 grams protein, 6.1 grams carbohydrate, 8.7 grams fat (1.3 saturated), 0 milligrams cholesterol, 91 milligrams sodium, 1.2 grams fibre

helpful hints

- *Shredded cabbage can be bought ready-to-eat in the fruit and veg section of some supermarkets.*
- *Crumbled feta cheese can be found in the dairy section of the supermarket.*
- *Dried oregano and dill are used in this recipe. Replace dried herbs after 6 months. If they look grey and old, that's probably how they will taste.*

countdown

- *Assemble salad.*
- *Make prawns.*

shopping list

FRUIT AND VEG

  1 bag shredded, washed,
    ready-to-eat cabbage

  1 bag shredded, washed,
    ready-to-eat cos lettuce

  1 small bunch spring onions

  1 large tomato

DAIRY

  1 small packet crumbled feta
    cheese

SEAFOOD

  350g (12oz) large prawns

STAPLES

  Olive oil and vinegar dressing

  Olive oil

  Frozen chopped onion

  Garlic

  Dried dill

  Dried oregano

  Salt

  Black peppercorns

helpful hints

- There are several jerk seasonings, liquid and dry, available. Choose whichever one suits your taste.
- If jerk seasoning is unavailable, make your own by mixing 1 teaspoon dried thyme, 1 teaspoon salt, $\frac{1}{2}$ teaspoon allspice, $\frac{1}{2}$ teaspoon cinnamon and a pinch of cayenne pepper together.
- If you are really pressed for time, serve the jerk pork with a washed, ready-to eat salad and 2 tablespoons of no-sugar-added salad dressing instead of the palm heart salad.

countdown

- Assemble salad.
- Make Jerk Pork.

shopping list

FRUIT AND VEG
  1 bag washed, ready-to-eat salad
  1 medium cucumber
  2 medium tomatoes
MEAT
  2 x 175g (6oz) boneless pork chops
GROCERY
  400g (14oz) tin palm hearts
  1 small bottle jerk seasoning
STAPLES
  No-sugar-added oil and vinegar dressing
  Rapeseed oil

jamaican jerk pork

This meal fits the nutritional guidelines for the Quick Start phase.

'Jerking' is an ancient Jamaican method for preserving and cooking meat. In Jamaica the men who prepare the meat and sell it to the markets are called 'jerk men'. They use a long process involving marinating the meat and then slowly cooking it over a pimiento (allspice) wood fire. I've captured the flavours of jerk cooking for this quick dinner by using a prepared jerk seasoning.

jamaican jerk pork

2 x 175g (6oz) boneless pork chops, about 1cm ($\frac{1}{2}$in) thick
1 tablespoon jerk seasoning
1 teaspoon rapeseed oil

Remove fat from pork and rub with jerk seasoning. Heat oil in a medium-sized non-stick frying pan on medium-high heat. Add pork and brown for 2 minutes. Turn and brown second side for 2 minutes. Lower heat to medium and cook 2 more minutes. A meat thermometer should read 70ºC/160ºC. Makes 2 servings.
Makes 2 servings.

Per serving: 287 calories, 45.3 grams protein, 1.5 grams carbohydrate, 9.8 grams fat (3.0 saturated), 146 milligrams cholesterol, 107 milligrams sodium, 0 grams fibre

palm heart salad

400g (14oz) tin palm hearts
150g (5oz) washed, ready-to-eat salad
$\frac{1}{2}$ medium cucumber, peeled and sliced
2 tablespoons no-sugar-added oil and vinegar dressing
2 medium tomatoes, quartered

Drain palm hearts and cut into 2.5cm (1in) slices. Place prepared salad in a bowl and add cucumber and dressing. Toss well. Add tomato wedges along edge of bowl and sprinkle palm hearts on top.
Makes 2 servings.

Per serving: 160 calories, 6.8 grams protein, 15.9 grams carbohydrate, 9.5 grams fat (1.4 saturated), 0 milligrams cholesterol, 715 milligrams sodium, 4.3 grams fibre

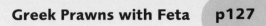
Greek Prawns with Feta   p127

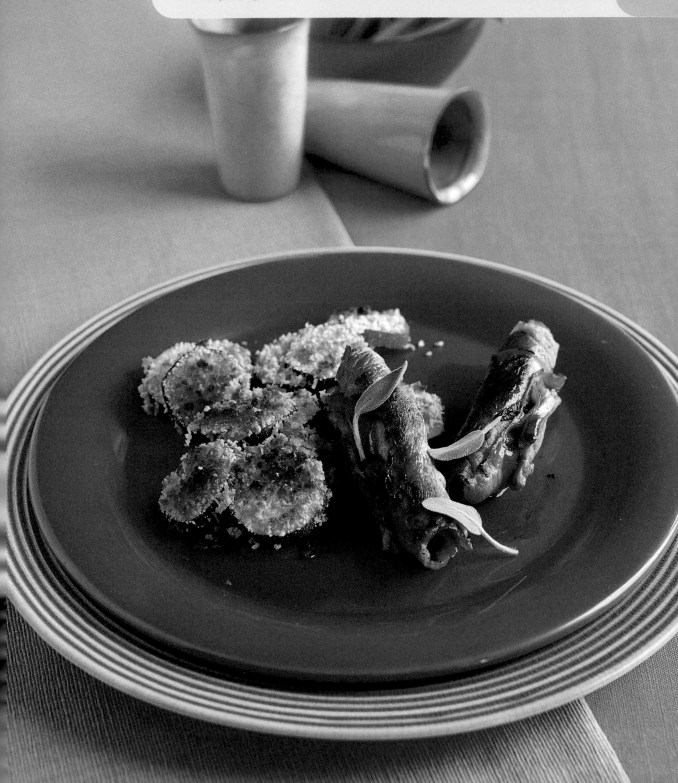

Savory Sage Chicken with Italian Zucchini and Tomatoes   **p129**

savoury sage chicken

This is a tasty, 10-minute meal created by adding a quick sage and flour coating and a wine sauce to shop-bought roasted chicken.

savoury sage chicken

1 tablespoon flour

2 teaspoons dried ground sage

Salt and freshly ground black pepper

2 x 175g (6oz) roasted boneless, skinless chicken breasts

1 tablespoon olive oil

50ml (2fl oz) dry vermouth

50ml (2fl oz) water

Mix together flour, sage and salt and pepper to taste. Roll chicken in mixture, pressing flour into chicken on both sides. Heat a medium-sized non-stick frying pan on medium-high heat. Add chicken to pan and cook for 1 minute per side. Remove to a plate and raise heat to high. Add vermouth and water and reduce for 2 minutes. Pour sauce over chicken.

Makes 2 servings.

Per serving: 383 calories, 54.5 grams protein, 4.1 grams carbohydrate, 14.9 grams fat (2.7 saturated), 144 milligrams cholesterol, 131 milligrams sodium, 0 grams fibre

italian courgettes and tomatoes

110g (4oz) courgettes, sliced

2 medium tomatoes, cut into wedges about same size as courgettes

1 teaspoon dried oregano

2 tablespoons grated semi-skimmed milk mozzarella cheese

Salt and freshly ground black pepper

Place courgettes and tomatoes in a microwave-safe bowl and microwave on high for 3 minutes. Add oregano, cheese and salt and pepper to taste. Toss well.

Makes 2 servings.

Per serving: 74 calories, 6.5 grams protein, 9.6 grams carbohydrate, 2.1 grams fat (1.2 saturated), 7 milligrams cholesterol, 67 milligrams sodium, 0.9 grams fibre

helpful hints

● *White wine can be substituted for vermouth.*

● *Roasted boneless, skinless chicken breasts come ready packaged in the the supermarket. Or use rotisserie-roasted chicken breasts.*

● *Dried oregano and sage are used in this recipe. Replace dried herbs after 6 months. If they look grey and old, that's probably how they will taste.*

countdown

● *Make Italian Courgettes and Tomatoes.*

● *Make Savoury Sage Chicken.*

shopping list

FRUIT AND VEG

110g (4oz) courgettes

2 medium tomatoes

DAIRY

1 small packet grated semi-skimmed milk mozzarella cheese

MEAT

2 X 175g (6oz) roasted boneless, skinless chicken breasts

GROCERY

1 small bottle dry vermouth

STAPLES

Dried oregano

Dried ground sage

Flour

Olive oil

Salt

Black peppercorns

which carb

super speed

suppers

swordfish in spanish sofrito sauce

This meal fits the nutritional guidelines for the Which Carbs phase.

Onions, garlic, green peppers and tomatoes form the basis for a Spanish sofrito sauce. The Italian sofrito is similar using chopped celery, green peppers, onion, garlic and herbs. It's used for soups and stews. Spanish sofrito can be bought in a jar or tin in some supermarkets. If difficult to find, use a thick tomato salsa instead.

Brown rice takes about 45 minutes to cook. There are several brands of quick-cooking brown rice available. Their cooking time ranges from 10 to 30 minutes. The 10-minute rice is used in this dinner.

swordfish in spanish sofrito sauce

350g (12oz) swordfish
2 teaspoons olive oil
Salt and freshly ground black
    pepper
225ml (8fl oz) sofrito or thick no-
    sugar-added tomato salsa

Wash fish and pat dry with kitchen paper. Heat oil in a medium-sized non-stick frying pan on medium-high heat and add fish. Brown for 2 minutes. Turn and brown second side for 2 minutes. Season cooked sides with salt and pepper. Lower heat to medium, add sofrito, cover, and simmer for 5 minutes for 2.5cm (1in) thick fish, 3–4 minutes for 1.5cm ($\frac{1}{2}$ in) thick fish.
Makes 2 servings.

> Per serving: 308 calories, 33.6 grams protein, 0 grams carbohydrate, 12.8 grams fat (2.4 saturated), 66 milligrams cholesterol, 152 milligrams sodium, 0 grams fibre

yellow rice

300ml (11fl oz) water
300ml (11fl oz) 10-minute quick-
    cooking brown rice
$\frac{1}{2}$ teaspoon turmeric
50g (2oz) diced or sliced sweet
    pepper, drained
1 teaspoon olive oil

Bring water to the boil in a large saucepan over high heat. Lower heat to medium-high and add rice. Cover and cook for 5 minutes. Remove from heat and let stand for 5 minutes. Stir in pimiento and olive oil. Add salt and pepper to taste.
Makes 2 servings.

> Per serving: 196 calories, 5.0 grams protein, 36.0 grams carbohydrate, 3.9 grams fat (0.6 saturated), 0 milligrams cholesterol, 3 milligrams sodium, 2 grams fibre

helpful hints

- *Any meaty fish such as halibut or tuna can be used. This meal also works well with tinned tuna.*
- *Saffron can be used instead of the turmeric in the rice.*
- *Look for: sofrito with 15 calories and 0.4 grams of fat per 25g (1oz).*

countdown

- *Start rice.*
- *Make swordfish.*
- *Assemble dessert.*

shopping list

SEAFOOD
    350g (12oz) swordfish
GROCERY
    *1 jar sofrito or thick no-sugar-
        added tomato salsa*
    1 small jar turmeric
    *1 small jar diced or sliced
        sweet pepper*
STAPLES
    Olive oil
    *10-minute quick-cooking
        brown rice*
    Salt
    Black peppercorns

peasant country soup

This meal fits the nutritional guidelines for the Which Carbs phase.

This warm, hearty soup can be made in about 15 minutes. It keeps well. Make extra and freeze for another quick meal if you have the time.

peasant country soup

2 teaspoons olive oil
450g (1lb) sliced button
   mushrooms
350ml (12fl oz) pasta sauce
175ml (6fl oz) fat-free, low-sodium
   chicken stock
175ml (6fl oz) water
175g (6oz) cooked white haricot
   or cannellini beans, rinsed and
   drained
110g (4oz) roasted chicken strips
   or pieces
Salt and freshly ground black
   pepper

Heat olive oil in a medium-sized saucepan over high heat. Add mushrooms and sauté for 1 minute. Add pasta sauce, chicken stock, water and beans. Bring to the boil and simmer for 10 minutes. Add chicken and cook for 1 minute to warm through. Add salt and pepper to taste.
Makes 2 servings.

> Per serving: 334 calories, 29.7 grams protein, 33.6 grams carbohydrate, 8.7 grams fat (1.2 saturated), 48 milligrams cholesterol, 856 milligrams sodium, 6.2 grams fibre

herb cheese toast and salad

2 slices wholemeal bread
Olive oil spray
50g (2oz) herbed goat cheese
150g (5oz) washed, ready-to-
   serve salad
2 tablespoons no-sugar-added oil
   and vinegar dressing

Pre-heat grill. Spray wholemeal slices with olive oil spray and spread with goat cheese. Grill for 1 to 2 minutes until cheese is melted. Cut bread into 2 triangles. Place salad in a bowl and toss with dressing. Divide between 2 salad plates and place 2 toast triangles (1 slice) on the side. Serve with soup.
Makes 2 servings.

> Per serving: 237 calories, 10.7 grams protein, 12.6 grams carbohydrate, 18.0 grams fat (7.1 saturated), 22 milligrams cholesterol, 342 milligrams sodium, 3.3 grams fibre

helpful hints

- Buy thin sliced mushrooms in the fruit and veg section of the supermarket.
- Any type of tinned beans can be used.

countdown

- Pre-heat grill.
- Make soup.
- Make Herb Cheese Toast and Salad.

shopping list

FRUIT AND VEG
   450g (1lb) sliced button
      mushrooms
   1 bag washed, ready-to-serve
      salad
DAIRY
   50g (2oz) herbed goat cheese
MEAT
   110g (4oz) roasted chicken
      strips or pieces
STAPLES:
   Fat-free, low-sodium chicken
      stock
   Olive oil
   Olive oil spray
   Wholemeal bread
   No-sugar-added oil and
      vinegar dressing
   No-sugar-added, pasta sauce
      (350ml/12fl oz needed)
   White haricot or cannellini
      beans
   Salt
   Black peppercorns

beef teriyaki with chinese noodles

This meal fits the nutritional guidelines for the Which Carbs phase.

Juicy beef in a spicy teriyaki sauce is a traditional Japanese dish. This one can be made in minutes by buying the teriyaki sauce and the vegetables already cut for stir-fry. Some supermarkets have the meat and vegetables cut and ready to use for stir-frying in one packet. Or go to the salad bar section and buy the vegetables cut up there.

beef teriyaki

350g (12oz) sirloin steak, cut for stir-fry
1 teaspoon sesame oil
225g (8oz) sliced onion
2 garlic cloves, crushed
110g (4oz) sliced mushrooms
50ml (2fl oz) teriyaki sauce

Cut beef into strips, 7.5cm (3in) long and 0.5cm (¼in) wide, if not already cut. Heat sesame oil in a non-stick frying pan or wok on high heat. Add onion, garlic and mushrooms. Stir-fry for 2 minutes. Add beef and stir-fry for 1 minute. Add teriyaki sauce and continue to cook for 1 minute. *Makes 2 servings.*

Per serving: 456 calories, 63.9 grams protein, 14.2 grams carbohydrate, 17.3 grams fat (7.6 saturated), 153 milligrams cholesterol, 755 milligrams sodium, 0 grams fibre

chinese noodles

110g (4oz) fresh Chinese noodles or dried noodles
1 teaspoon sesame oil
6 spring onions, sliced
Salt and freshly ground black pepper

Bring 2–3 litres (4–5 pints) of water to the boil in a large saucepan over high heat. Add noodles and cook for 1 minute or according to packet instructions. Drain. Add sesame oil, spring onions and salt and pepper to taste. Divide between 2 dinner plates and serve Beef Teriyaki on top.
Makes 2 servings.

Per serving: 167 calories, 5.0 grams protein, 27.6 grams carbohydrate, 4.0 grams fat (0.6 saturated), 33 milligrams cholesterol, 9 milligrams sodium, 1.1 grams fibre

helpful hints

- *Look out for 'light' teriyaki sauce with 15 calories per tablespoon, 320 mg sodium and 3 grams carbohydrates.*
- *Rapeseed oil can be used instead of sesame oil.*
- *Fresh Chinese noodles can be found in the fruit and veg section of the supermarket. Or dried noodles can be used.*
- *Angel-hair pasta can be substituted for the Chinese noodles.*
- *Beef topside can be used instead of sirloin.*

countdown

- *Boil water for noodles.*
- *Make Beef Teriyaki.*
- *Make Chinese Noodles.*

shopping list

FRUIT AND VEG
1 small packet sliced mushrooms (110g/ 4oz needed)
1 small bunch spring onions
1 small packet fresh Chinese noodles or dried noodles
MEAT
350g (12oz) sirloin steak, cut for stir-fry
GROCERY
1 small bottle sesame oil
1 small bottle teriyaki sauce
STAPLES
Onion
Garlic
Salt
Black peppercorns

right carb

super speed

lunches

parmesan sole

This meal fits the nutritional guidelines for the Right Carbs phase.

Fish is the original fast food. It takes only minutes to cook. For this quick meal, grated Parmesan cheese and breadcrumbs top the sole. This entire meal can be put together in 15 minutes.

parmesan sole

Olive oil spray
350g (12oz) sole fillet (1cm/½in thick)
2 teaspoons olive oil
2 tablespoons plain breadcrumbs
2 tablespoons freshly grated Parmesan cheese
Salt and freshly ground black pepper
2 small tomatoes, sliced

Pre-heat grill. Line a baking tray with foil and spray with olive oil spray. Rinse fish and pat dry. Place on tray and brush with 1 teaspoon olive oil. Grill for 5 minutes. Mix together breadcrumbs, Parmesan cheese, remaining oil and salt and pepper to taste. Remove sole from grill and place tomato slices over fish. Spread breadcrumb mixture evenly over fish. Grill for 2 minutes. Remove and serve.
Makes 2 servings.

> Per serving: 287 calories, 38.1 grams protein, 6.8 grams carbohydrate, 11.5 grams fat (3.4 saturated), 64 milligrams cholesterol, 300 milligrams sodium, 0 grams fibre

potato cubes

350g (12oz) new potatoes
2 teaspoons olive oil
Salt and freshly ground black pepper

Wash, but do not peel, potatoes. Cut into 2.5cm (1in) cubes. Place in a microwave-safe bowl and cover with clingfilm or a plate. Microwave on high for 5 minutes. Remove and let stand, covered, for 1 minute. Remove cover carefully, because the steam will be very hot. Add olive oil and salt and pepper to taste. Toss well.
Makes 2 servings.

> Per serving: 180 calories, 3.5 grams protein, 30.6 grams carbohydrate, 4.7 grams fat (0.6 saturated), 0 milligrams cholesterol, 11 milligrams sodium, 2.7 grams fibre

dessert

450g (1lb) melon cubes

Divide between 2 dessert bowls.
Makes 2 servings.

> Per serving: 86 calories, 2.1 grams protein, 20.1 grams carbohydrate, 0.6 grams fat (0 saturated), 0 milligrams cholesterol, 21 milligrams sodium, 0.8 grams fibre

helpful hints

- *Any type of delicate white fish fillet can be used such as snapper or flounder.*
- *Fresh melon cubes can be found in the fruit and veg section of most supermarkets.*

countdown

- *Pre-heat grill.*
- *Make potato cubes.*
- *Make Parmesan Sole.*
- *Assemble dessert.*

shopping list

FRUIT AND VEG
  350g (12oz) new potatoes
  2 small tomatoes
  1 container melon cubes (about 450g/1lb)
SEAFOOD
  350g (12oz) sole fillet
GROCERY
  Plain breadcrumbs
STAPLES
  Olive oil spray
  Olive oil
  Parmesan cheese
  Salt
  Black peppercorns

chicken creole

This meal fits the nutritional guidelines for the Right Carbs phase.

Green pepper and onions are essential ingredients of Creole and Cajun cooking. Add some tomatoes, hot peppers and chicken and you've got a quick and easy Chicken Creole. The amount of cayenne called for in the recipe gives a mild zing to the sauce. If you like it hot, add more cayenne or serve hot pepper sauce at the table.

Brown rice takes about 45 minutes to cook. There are several brands of quick-cooking brown rice available. Their cooking time ranges from 10 to 30 minutes. The 10-minute rice is used in this recipe.

helpful hints

● Look for roasted chicken breasts that have not been cooked in a honey, sugar or barbecue sauce.

● Dried oregano is used in this recipe. Replace dried herbs after 6 months. If they look grey and old, that's probably how they will taste.

● Fresh watermelon cubes can be found in the fruit and veg section of some supermarkets.

countdown

● Boil water for rice.

● Make chicken dish and cover to keep warm.

● Make rice.

● Assemble the dessert.

chicken creole

1 teaspoon olive oil

350g (12oz) frozen chopped onion

225g (8oz) frozen diced green pepper

4 garlic cloves, crushed

450g (1lb) no-sugar-added chopped tomatoes

2 teaspoons dried oregano

1 tablespoon Worcestershire sauce

1/8 teaspoon cayenne pepper

350g (12oz) roasted boneless, skinless chicken breast, cut into 2.5cm (1in) cubes

Salt and freshly ground black pepper

Hot pepper sauce

Heat olive oil in a medium-sized non-stick frying pan on medium-high heat and add onion, green pepper and garlic. Sauté for 2 minutes. Add tomatoes, oregano, Worcestershire sauce, cayenne pepper and chicken to pan. Simmer for 3 minutes. Add salt and pepper to taste. Spoon chicken and sauce over rice and pass the hot pepper sauce.

Makes 2 servings.

Per serving: 436 calories, 59.1 grams protein, 28.1 grams carbohydrate, 10.5 grams fat (2.2 saturated), 144 milligrams cholesterol, 411 milligrams sodium, 4.6 grams fibre

quick brown rice

175g (6oz) 10-minute quick-
cooking brown rice
225ml (8fl oz) water
Salt and freshly ground black
pepper

Bring water to the boil in a large saucepan over high heat and add rice. Boil for 5 minutes. Cover with a lid and let stand for 5 minutes. Or follow packet instructions. Fluff with a fork and add salt and pepper to taste.
Makes 2 servings.

Per serving: 128 calories, 3.8 grams protein, 26.3 grams carbohydrate, 1.3 grams fat (0.2 saturated), 0 milligrams cholesterol, 0 milligrams sodium, 1.5 grams fibre

dessert

275g (10oz) watermelon cubes

Divide between 2 dessert bowls.
Makes 2 servings.

Per serving: 49 calories, 1 gram protein, 11.1 grams carbohydrate, 0.7 grams fat (0.1 saturated), 0 milligrams cholesterol, 3 milligrams sodium, 0.8 grams fibre

shopping list

FRUIT AND VEG
  275g (10oz) watermelon
    cubes
MEAT
  350g (12oz) roasted
    boneless, skinless chicken
    breast
GROCERY
  450g (1lb) tin no-sugar-
    added chopped tomatoes
STAPLES
  Frozen chopped onion
  Frozen diced green pepper
  Garlic
  Cayenne pepper
  Dried oregano
  Worcestershire sauce
  Hot pepper sauce
  10-minute, quick-cooking
    brown rice
  Olive oil
  Salt
  Black peppercorns

black bean soup with rice

helpful hints

● If you like your black bean soup thick, remove about 110g (4oz) of beans from the soup after it is cooked and purée them in a food processor. Stir the purée into the soup.

● Any type of hard grating cheese can be used.

● Brown rice takes about 45 minutes to cook. There are several brands of quick-cooking brown rice available. Their cooking time ranges from 10 to 30 minutes. Use the 10-minute rice for this dinner.

countdown

● Make rice.
● Make soup.

shopping list

DAIRY
  1 small packet Manchego cheese
DELI
  175g (6oz) lean gammon
STAPLES
  10-minute, quick-cooking brown rice
  Chilli powder
  Frozen chopped onion
  Frozen diced green pepper
  Olive oil
  Tinned black beans (225g/ 8oz needed)
  Fat-free, low-sodium chicken stock
  Salt
  Black peppercorns

This meal fits the nutritional guidelines for the Right Carbs phase.

This hearty black bean soup makes a quick one-pot dinner. Manchego is a flavourful, semi-firm Spanish cheese made from sheep's milk.

rice

110g (4oz) 10-minute quick-cooking brown rice
150ml (5fl oz) water
Salt and freshly ground black pepper

Bring water to the boil in a large saucepan over high heat and add rice. Boil for 5 minutes. Cover with a lid and let stand for 5 minutes. Or follow packet instructions. Fluff with a fork and add salt and pepper to taste.

Makes 2 servings.

Per serving: 85 calories, 2.5 grams protein, 17.5 grams carbohydrate, 0.8 grams fat (0.2 saturated), 0 milligrams cholesterol, 0 milligrams sodium, 1 gram fibre

black bean soup

1 tablespoon olive oil
175g (6oz) lean gammon, cut into 5cm (2in) strips
225g (8oz) frozen diced green pepper
225g (8oz) frozen chopped onion
225g (8oz) rinsed and drained black beans
225ml (8fl oz) fat-free, low-sodium chicken stock
225ml (8fl oz) water
1 tablespoon chilli powder
Salt and freshly ground black pepper
50g (2oz) grated Manchego cheese

Heat olive oil in a large saucepan on medium-high heat. Add the gammon, green pepper and onion. Sauté for 1 minute. Add beans, chicken stock, water and chilli powder. Bring to a simmer and cook for 5 minutes. Add salt and pepper to taste. Sprinkle cheese on top. To serve, divide rice between 2 soup bowls and spoon soup on top.

Makes 2 servings.

Per serving: 555 calories, 41.8 grams protein, 54.0 grams carbohydrate, 19.4 grams fat (6.9 saturated), 65 milligrams cholesterol, 1100 milligrams sodium, 7.2 grams fibre

mock hungarian goulash

This meal fits the nutritional guidelines for the Right Carbs phase.

Succulent beef in a tomato sauce flavoured with onion, green pepper and paprika is the basis for Hungarian goulash. I've shortened this recipe by using good-quality, lean deli roast beef and called it Mock Hungarian Goulash. The secret to a good Hungarian goulash is good Hungarian paprika. Paprika is the Hungarian name for both sweet pepper and the powder made from it. Ordinary paprika comes in varying degrees of flavour – from pungent to virtually tasteless. True Hungarian paprika may be hot or mild and can be found in most supermarkets.

mock hungarian goulash

1 teaspoon olive oil

110g (4oz) frozen chopped onion

225g (8oz) frozen diced green pepper

40g (1¹/₂oz) sliced portobello mushrooms

1 tablespoon Hungarian paprika or 1¹/₂ tablespoons paprika

225ml (8fl oz) low-sodium, no-sugar-added tomato sauce

175g (6oz) thick sliced lean deli roast beef, cut into 1cm (¹/₂in) wide strips

Salt and freshly ground black pepper

2 tablespoons reduced-fat crème fraiche

2 medium tomatoes, cut into wedges

Heat oil in a medium-sized non-stick frying pan on medium-high heat and add onion, green pepper and mushrooms. Sauté for 1 minute. Sprinkle paprika over vegetables and sauté for 3 minutes. Add tomato sauce and simmer for 1 minute. Add roast beef and salt and pepper to taste. Remove from heat and serve over noodles. Spoon crème fraiche on top and arrange tomatoes on the side.
Makes 2 servings.

Per serving: 311 calories, 31.0 grams protein, 21.3 grams carbohydrate, 10.8 grams fat (4.0 saturated), 77 milligrams cholesterol, 100 milligrams sodium, 1.5 grams fibre

caraway noodles

110g (4oz) flat egg noodles

2 teaspoons olive oil

1 tablespoon caraway seeds

Salt and freshly ground black pepper

Bring 2–3 litres (4–5 pints) of water to the boil in a large saucepan over high heat. Add the noodles and boil for 3–4 minutes or according to packet instructions. Drain, leaving about 2 tablespoons water with the noodles. Toss with oil and caraway seeds. Add salt and pepper to taste. Divide between 2 plates and spoon goulash on top.
Makes 2 servings.

Per serving: 228 calories, 6.7 grams protein, 34.8 grams carbohydrate, 6.6 grams fat (1.0 saturated), 46 milligrams cholesterol, 10 milligrams sodium, 1.5 grams fibre

helpful hints

● *Look for thinly sliced mushrooms in the fruit and veg section of the supermarket. Any type of sliced mushrooms can be used.*

● *If Hungarian paprika is unavailable, use regular paprika. If you have it on hand, make sure it is a fresh jar. If your paprika is older than 6 months, it's time for a fresh jar.*

countdown

● *Boil water for noodles.*
● *Make goulash.*
● *Make noodles.*

shopping list

FRUIT AND VEG
   1 small packet sliced portobello mushrooms (about 40g/1¹/₂oz needed)
   2 medium tomatoes
DAIRY
   1 small pot reduced-fat crème fraiche
DELI
   175g (6oz) thick-sliced lean deli roast beef
GROCERY
   1 jar Hungarian paprika or ordinary paprika
   1 small jar caraway seeds
   110g (4oz) flat egg noodles
STAPLES
   Olive oil
   Frozen chopped onion
   Frozen diced green pepper
   Low-sodium, no-sugar-added tomato sauce
   Salt
   Black peppercorns

weekends

By noon on Fridays, I'm already looking forward to relaxing over the weekend and spending time with my family. I also look forward to meals on which I make a little extra effort, to make them special, but I don't want to slave over the stove all day preparing them. The recipes are full of flavour and intrigue. Just who could resist the idea of Spiced Cowboy Steak with Jalapeño Rice? Puts you into a good mood for watching a great movie on Saturday night. Though the rice does take a little time to cook, it doesn't involve you in a lot of work.

How to manage a blow-out weekend? No need to worry here. Remember, balance is the key. My husband has never found it difficult, even after a deviation, to return to the low-carb lifestyle, because the menus are so appealing and varied. Seasonal eating is ever-important. You will want fresh fish and light pasta dishes and salads in summer when the supermarket shelves are filled with a huge array of saladings and vibrantly coloured peppers, squashes and sweet vine-ripened tomatoes. In winter the more robust meats and hearty cabbage dishes provide warming, comfort food to tempt you to stay with the low-carb lifestyle.

The recipes in this section are still quick and easy, but they take a few extra minutes of preparation or contain special ingredients that you may not think of for week-night dinners. I've often made dinner party menus using these dishes and been asked for the recipes!

Garlic-Stuffed Steak is a fun weekend meal that meets the guidelines for the Quick Start section.

Chicken and Walnuts in Lettuce Puffs is a dinner with an Asian theme that fits the Which Carb Meal Plan. Asian flavours are all the rage now that we travel so much more widely in countries such as Laos, Vietnam and Korea, and chefs in the West are experimenting with fusion dishes which can often be easily adapted to low-carb eating. The secret of staying with a low-carb lifestyle is providing enough variation in one's diet to satisfy the taste buds. Don't get bored or you may be tempted to stray.

Pan-Seared Tuna with Mango Salsa is a delightful blend of fusion flavours and styles that fits the Right Carbs phase. There is the opportunity to mix and match, but the meals have been created to achieve the nutritional priorities of that phase in your diet. My husband and I no longer think about what is and what isn't low-carb; we just consider it good food that fits into our busy schedules and is appreciated by our families.

And of course you can have desserts. Pears with Raspberry Coulis makes a refreshing end to a great Saturday evening feast.

All of the weekend meals in this section are incorporated in the 2-week plan for the appropriate phase.

quick start
weekend
m e a l s

dijon chicken with crunchy couscous

The nutritional analysis for this recipes fits the Quick Start phase.

A tangy mustard sauce gently coats these chicken breasts. The couscous is made with lettuce, giving a crunchy texture to the couscous. We don't often think of cooking lettuce, but the French braise lettuce and use it to make soup.

dijon chicken

2 x 175g (6oz) boneless, skinless chicken breasts

Olive oil spray

Freshly ground black pepper

115ml (4fl oz) dry vermouth

2 tablespoons Dijon mustard

2 tablespoons coarse-grain mustard

1 tablespoon whipping cream

Place chicken between 2 pieces of greaseproof paper and flatten with a kitchen mallet or the bottom of a heavy pan to 1cm (½in) thick. Heat a medium-sized non-stick frying pan on medium-high heat and spray with olive oil spray. Brown chicken for 2 minutes, then turn and brown second side for 2 minutes. Season the cooked sides with pepper to taste. Remove chicken to a plate and add vermouth to the pan. Cook for 30 seconds, then add the two mustards and stir to blend, about 30 seconds. Return chicken to the pan and cook for 1 minute. Remove pan from heat and stir in the cream. Sprinkle over pepper to taste. Serve chicken on 2 dinner plates with the sauce spooned on top. *Makes 2 servings.*

> Per serving: 400 calories, 55.4 grams protein, 3.7 grams carbohydrate, 14.2 grams fat (4.2 saturated), 155 milligrams cholesterol, 859 milligrams sodium, 0 grams fibre

crunchy couscous

225ml (8fl oz) water

110g (4oz) pre-cooked couscous

175g (6oz) shredded iceberg lettuce

Salt and freshly ground black pepper

2 tablespoons flaked almonds

Several sprigs watercress, for garnish

Bring water to the boil in a medium saucepan on high heat. Add couscous and lettuce. Remove from the heat, cover, and let sit for 5 minutes. Fluff couscous with a fork and add almonds and salt and pepper to taste. Arrange sprigs of watercress on the side. *Makes 2 servings.*

> Per serving: 146 calories, 5.8 grams protein, 18.4 grams carbohydrate, 6.2 grams fat (0.4 saturated), 0 milligrams cholesterol, 12 milligrams sodium, 2.1 grams fibre

helpful hints

- Four tablespoons of Dijon mustard can be used instead of the combination of Dijon and coarse-grain mustard.
- Any type of berry can be used for the dessert.
- Look for low-fat frozen yoghurt with 240 calories, 6 grams fat and 40 grams carbs per 225ml (8fl oz). Some brands have fewer calories and less fat and carbs. Use whichever one you can find.

countdown

- Make couscous.
- Make chicken.
- Assemble the dessert just before serving.

shopping list

FRUIT AND VEG

1 small head iceberg lettuce

1 bunch watercress

DAIRY

1 small pot whipping cream

MEAT

2 x 175g (6oz) boneless, skinless chicken breasts

GROCERY

1 small bottle dry vermouth

1 small jar coarse-grain mustard

1 small packet couscous

1 small packet flaked almonds

STAPLES

Olive oil spray

Dijon mustard

Salt

Black peppercorns

garlic-stuffed steak

The nutritional analysis for this recipes fits the Quick Start phase.
Garlic and parsley stuffed into a juicy steak make a perfect quick meal for the weekend.

The garlic cloves for this stuffing are blanched first and then chopped with fresh parsley to make a simple stuffing. Blanching gives the garlic a mild, sweet flavour. The water used for blanching the garlic has a wonderful flavour, so I add it to the water for cooking the pasta.

The asparagus is added for the last 5 minutes to the boiling pasta. This saves time and an extra pot to wash. If using fresh pasta, the cooking time will be about 3–4 minutes. Add the asparagus first and then the fresh pasta.

helpful hints

- Any type of quick-cooking steak such as sirloin or fillet can be used.
- Use the same pan for boiling pasta and garlic to save clean-up time.
- The blanched garlic and parsley can be chopped in a food processor.
- Buy good-quality Parmesan cheese and grate it yourself or chop it in the food processor. Freeze extra for quick use. You can quickly spoon out what you need and leave the rest frozen.

countdown

- Blanch garlic and then fill the pan with more water and place on heat to boil.
- Make steak.
- Make linguine and asparagus.

shopping list

FRUIT AND VEG
  1 medium tomato
  1 small head romaine lettuce
DELI
  110g (4oz) smoked turkey
STAPLES
  Eggs (6 needed)
  Parmesan cheese
  Salt
  Black peppercorns

garlic-stuffed steak

5 garlic cloves, peeled
350g (12oz) frying steak
15g (1oz) chopped parsley
Salt and freshly ground black pepper
1 teaspoon olive oil

Place whole, peeled garlic cloves in a large saucepan and cover with cold water. Bring to the boil and scoop out garlic cloves with a strainer. Fill the saucepan with more cold water and bring to the boil for the pasta side dish.

Remove fat from steak and make slits about 2.5cm (1in) apart on top and bottom to form pockets for the stuffing. The slits should be about 1cm (½in) deep and cover the width of the steak.

Chop the garlic and parsley together. Add salt and pepper to taste. With the tip of a knife or a small spoon, stuff the slits in the steak using about half the parsley mixture. Set the rest of the stuffing aside. Heat a medium-sized non-stick frying pan on medium-high heat and add the stuffed steak. Sauté for 5 minutes. Turn and sauté 5 minutes for rare. A meat thermometer should read 60ºC/145ºF degrees. Cook 1–2 minutes longer for medium rare, or longer if you prefer your meat more well cooked. Season the cooked sides of steak. Remove from the frying pan to a chopping board and add the olive oil to the pan. Add remaining stuffing and sauté for 1–2 minutes. Cut the steak into 2.5cm (1in) slices and divide between 2 dinner plates. Spoon sautéed stuffing on top of slices.
Makes 2 servings.

Per serving: 397 calories, 61.5 grams protein, 3.6 grams carbohydrate, 17.1 grams fat (7.5 saturated), 153 milligrams cholesterol, 119 milligrams sodium, 0 grams fibre

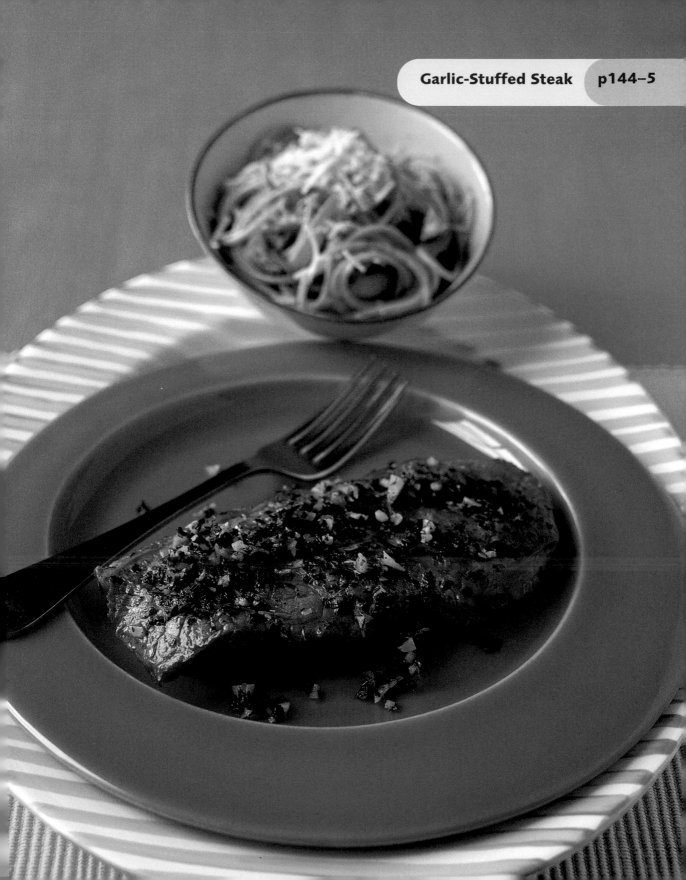

Garlic-Stuffed Steak   p144–5

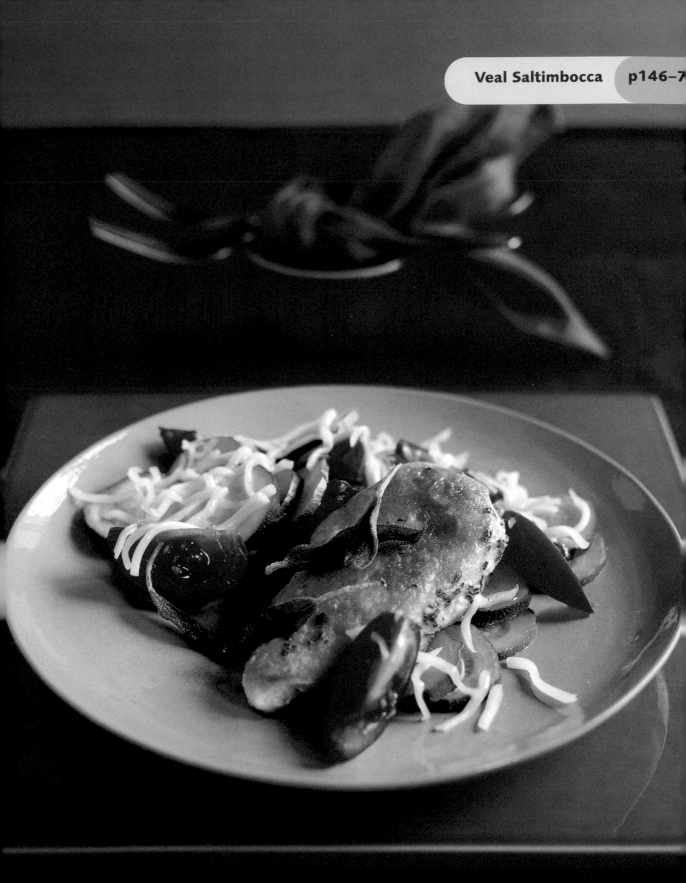

linguine and asparagus

50g (2oz) wholemeal linguine
110g (4oz) asparagus
2 teaspoons olive oil
*Salt and freshly ground black
   pepper*
*2 tablespoons grated Parmesan
   cheese*

Bring a large saucepan with 2–3 litres (4–5 pints) of water to the boil on high heat, using the garlic water from the stuffed steak recipe and additional water to make up the quantity. Add the pasta and boil for 5 minutes. Cut 2.5cm (1in) from bottom of asparagus end and cut the asparagus spears into 2.5cm (1in) slices. Add the asparagus to the pasta and continue to boil for 5 minutes. Remove 2 tablespoons of the water and place in a large bowl. Drain the pasta and asparagus. Add olive oil and salt and pepper to taste to the water in the bowl. Add the drained pasta and toss well. Sprinkle with Parmesan cheese.
Makes 2 servings.

Per serving: 179 calories, 8.7 grams protein, 20.4 grams carbohydrate, 7.9 grams fat (2.5 saturated), 7 milligrams cholesterol, 180 milligrams sodium, 4.3 grams fibre

helpful hints

● *Any herb can be used.*
● *Dried tarragon is called for in the recipe. If using dried herbs, make sure the jar is less than 6 months old.*
● *For best results, use a good-quality non-stick pan.*

countdown

● *Prepare ingredients.*
● *Complete omelette.*

shopping list

FRUIT AND VEG
   110g (4oz) asparagus
   1 small bunch parsley
MEAT
   350g (12oz) frying steak
GROCERY
   1 small packet wholemeal linguine (50g/2oz needed)
STAPLES
   Garlic
   Olive oil
   Parmesan cheese
   Salt
   Black peppercorns

veal saltimbocca

The nutritional analysis for this recipes fits the Quick Start phase.

Saltimbocca means 'jump in mouth', which perfectly describes this dish. Fresh veal escalopes, an Italian staple, need only a few minutes cooking in a light wine sauce to flavour them.

helpful hints

● Ask the butcher to flatten the veal for you. Or flatten it with the bottom of a heavy frying pan or kitchen mallet.
● Veal may come in smaller pieces. Fill and roll in same manner, dividing filling among the pieces.

countdown

● Make Parmesan Courgettes and Italian Salad
● Make Veal Saltimbocca.

veal saltimbocca

2 x 75g (3oz) veal escalopes
Salt and freshly ground black
    pepper
2 thin slices lean ham (25g/1oz)
4 small fresh sage leaves
2 teaspoons olive oil
50ml (2fl oz) dry white wine
2 tablespoons water

Place veal on chopping board and season the side facing upwards. Lay one piece of ham on each piece. Cut each sage leaf into strips and place evenly on the ham. Roll up from the narrow end and secure with a wooden cocktail stick.

Heat the oil in a medium-sized non-stick frying pan on medium-high heat. Add the veal rollups and sauté until brown on all sides, about 2 minutes per side. Add the wine, lower heat to medium, and gently simmer for 5 minutes. Remove veal to 2 dinner plates and remove the cocktail sticks. Add water to frying pan and reduce the liquid over high heat for 1 minute. Add salt and pepper to taste. Spoon sauce over veal.

Makes 2 servings.

Per serving: 263 calories, 25.2 grams protein,
0.4 grams carbohydrate, 14.3 grams fat(6.3 saturated),
82 milligrams cholesterol, 178 milligrams sodium,
0 grams fibre

parmesan courgettes

*2 tablespoons grated Parmesan
cheese*

40g (1½oz) plain breadcrumbs

*225g (8oz) courgettes, cut into
1cm (½in) slices*

1 teaspoon olive oil

*Salt and freshly ground black
pepper*

Pre-heat grill. Mix Parmesan cheese and
breadcrumbs together and set aside. Place
courgette slices in a shallow, microwave-safe
bowl, cover, and microwave on high for 3
minutes. (Or bring a small saucepan filled with
water to the boil. Add courgettes and boil for
3–4 minutes. Drain and place in shallow baking
dish.) Drizzle olive oil and salt and pepper to
taste over the courgettes. Sprinkle with
Parmesan mixture and place under grill for 1–2
minutes or until topping is golden.
Makes 2 servings.

Per serving: 128 calories, 5.2 grams protein,
12.2 grams carbohydrate, 5.8 grams fat
(2.3 saturated), 7 milligrams cholesterol,
281 milligrams sodium, 0.8 grams fibre

italian salad

*150g (5oz) washed, ready-to-eat
Italian-style salad leaves*

*2 tablespoons no-sugar-added oil
and balsamic vinegar dressing*

Place salad in a bowl and add dressing. Toss
well.
Makes 2 servings.

Per serving: 87 calories, 0.8 grams protein, 2.3 grams
carbohydrate, 8.5 grams fat (1.3 saturated),
0 milligrams cholesterol, 83 milligrams sodium,
0.4 grams fibre

shopping list

FRUIT AND VEG

 *1 bag washed, ready-to-eat
  Italian-style salad leaves*

 225g (8oz) courgettes

 *1 small bunch fresh sage
  leaves*

DELI

 *1 small packet lean ham
  (25g/1oz needed)*

MEAT

 2 x 75g (3oz) veal escalopes

GROCERY

 1 small bottle dry white wine

 *1 small packet plain
  breadcrumbs*

 *1 bottle no-sugar-added oil
  and balsamic vinegar
  dressing*

STAPLES

 Parmesan cheese

 Olive oil

 Salt

 Black peppercorns

which carb

weekend

meals

spiced cowboy steak

The nutritional analysis for this recipe fits the Which Carbs phase.

Texas cowboys working near the Rio Grande border loved their cowboy steaks flavoured with Mexican spices. The spice mixture forms a crisp coating over the steak, keeping the meat juicy with a burst of flavour.

Brown rice takes about 45 minutes to cook. There are several brands of quick-cooking brown rice available. Their cooking time ranges from 10 to 30 minutes. I find the 30-minute rice has more flavour, but any quick-cooking rice will work for this dinner.

spiced cowboy steak

1 teaspoon ground cumin
1 teaspoon ground ginger
1 teaspoon dried thyme
1/8 teaspoon cayenne pepper
2 medium garlic cloves, crushed
350g (12oz) sirloin steak, fat
   removed
Olive oil spray
Salt

Pre-heat grill. Line a baking tray with foil. Combine cumin, ginger, thyme, cayenne and garlic in a bowl. Remove fat from steak. Spoon spice mixture over both sides of steak and press in with the back of a spoon. Spray both sides of steak with olive oil spray. Leave for 15 minutes while you prepare the rice.

Place steak on baking tray under grill. Grill for 5 minutes. Turn and grill for 4–5 minutes for medium rare. A meat thermometer should read 60ºC/145ºF degrees for rare. Grill a minute longer for a steak about 2.5cm (1in) thick. Cook longer if you prefer your meat more well done. Sprinkle with salt to taste.
Makes 2 servings.

> Per serving: 350 calories, 55.8 grams protein, 1.2 grams carbohydrate, 15.5 grams fat (7.2 saturated), 140 milligrams cholesterol, 104 milligrams sodium, 0 grams fibre

jalapeño rice

75g (3oz) 30-minute quick-
   cooking brown rice
2 tablespoons olive oil and vinegar
   dressing
2 medium jalapeno peppers,
   seeded and chopped
2 spring onions, thinly sliced
Salt and freshly ground black
   pepper

Bring a large saucepan with 2–3 litres (4–5 pints) water to the boil. Add rice to the saucepan, stir once or twice, and let boil for 30 minutes. Alternatively, follow the cooking instructions on the rice packet. Reserve 3 tablespoons cooking liquid and place in a serving bowl. Add the dressing to the bowl. Add peppers and spring onions. Drain rice and add to bowl. Add salt and pepper to taste. Toss well.
Makes 2 servings.

> Per serving: 237 calories, 5.2 grams protein, 34.3 grams carbohydrate, 9.8 grams fat (1.5 saturated), 0 milligrams cholesterol, 80 milligrams sodium, 1.5 grams fibre

helpful hints

● *Any type of frying steak can be used.*

● *Dried thyme is used in this recipe. Replace dried herbs after 6 months. If they look grey and old, that's probably how they will taste.*

countdown

● *Pre-heat grill and place foil-lined baking tray on top shelf.*

● *Start rice.*

● *Mix spices and garlic and marinate steak.*

● *Prepare remaining ingredients.*

● *Grill steak.*

● *Finish rice.*

shopping list

FRUIT AND VEG
   2 medium jalapeño peppers
   1 small bunch spring onions
MEAT
   350g (12oz) sirloin steak
      (fillet or rump can be used)
GROCERY
   Ground ginger
STAPLES
   Ground cumin
   Dried thyme
   Cayenne pepper
   Garlic
   Olive oil spray
   30-minute quick-cooking
      brown rice
   Olive oil and vinegar dressing
   Salt
   Black peppercorns

mediterranean snapper with provençal salad

The nutritional analysis for this recipes fits the Which Carbs phase.

Sunny Provence with its abundance of fresh vegetables and herbs has a cuisine that is fragrant and simple.

The snapper recipe calls for one uncommon vegetable – fennel. It has a bulbous look, with wide, celery-like stems and bright green feathery leaves. It has a very light aniseed flavour. I used the feathery leaves as a garnish.

Pernod, an aniseed-flavoured liqueur, is a perfect partner with fennel. You can buy small miniature Pernod bottles or use a dry vermouth instead.

provençal salad

1 tablespoon red wine vinegar
1 teaspoon Dijon mustard
1 teaspoon olive oil
50ml (2fl oz) non-fat natural
   yoghurt
small head round lettuce,
   washed and dried
4 radishes, sliced
1 small green pepper, sliced
6 stoned green olives
2 small wholemeal rolls

Pre-heat oven to 180ºC/350ºF/gas mark 4. Mix vinegar and mustard together in a salad bowl. Add oil and mix well. Blend in yoghurt. Add lettuce, radishes, green pepper and olives. Toss well. Warm rolls in oven while fish cooks.
Makes 2 servings.

Per serving: 145 calories, 7.9 grams protein, 20.8 grams carbohydrate, 5.2 grams fat (0.5 saturated), 1 milligram cholesterol, 493 milligrams sodium, 3.6 grams fibre

helpful hints

● *Any type of light white fish can be used. Cook the fish for 10 minutes per 2.5cm (1in) of thickness.*
● *Any type of lettuce can be used for the salad.*
● *Two tablespoons of a no-sugar-added dressing can be used for the salad instead of the dressing in recipe.*
● *Cut off fennel stalks and slice using the thin slicing blade of a food processor or mandoline.*
● *A quick way to chop the fennel leaves is to snip them off the stalk with scissors.*

countdown

● *Make dessert*
● *Pre-heat oven to warm rolls.*
● *Make salad.*
● *Heat rolls.*
● *Make fish.*

mediterranean snapper

*350g (12oz) red snapper fillets
(about 1cm/¹/₂ in thick)*
1 small bulb fennel, sliced
2 teaspoons olive oil
2 medium garlic cloves, crushed
50ml (2fl oz) Pernod
2 tablespoons whipping cream
*Salt and freshly ground black
pepper*

Rinse the fish and pat dry with kitchen paper.
Remove top of fennel leaving only white bulb;
wash feathery leaves and chop 2 tablespoons of
leaves. Reserve some fennel ferns for garnish.
Wash the fennel bulb and thinly slice. Heat the
oil in a medium-sized non-stick frying pan over
medium-high heat. Add fennel slices and leaves
and garlic. Sauté for 3 minutes. Add fish and
cook for 4 minutes per side. Remove fish to a
plate and cover with foil to keep warm.
Add Pernod and reduce for 1 minute over high
heat. Stir in cream and salt and pepper to taste.
Spoon sauce with sliced fennel over snapper
and sprinkle fennel ferns on top.
Makes 2 servings.

Per serving: 374 calories, 35.3 grams protein,
1.5 grams carbohydrate, 12.8 grams fat
(4.5 saturated), 83 milligrams cholesterol,
114 milligrams sodium, 0 grams fibre

pears with raspberry coulis

110g (4oz) raspberries
*Artificial sweetener equivalent to
2 teaspoons sugar*
2 medium pears

Place raspberries and sweetener in the bowl of a
food processor and process until smooth. If you
do not have a food processor, press berries
through a sieve. Spoon sauce on to 2 dessert
plates. Cut pears in half and remove core. Cut
into slices and place on sauce.
Makes 2 servings.

Per serving: 129 calories, 1.3 grams protein,
32.7 grams carbohydrate, 1.1 grams fat (0 saturated),
0 milligrams cholesterol, 1 milligram sodium,
7 grams fibre

shopping list

FRUIT AND VEG
 1 small bulb fennel
 1 small head round lettuce
 1 small bunch radishes
 1 small green pepper
 2 medium pears
 1 small punnet raspberries
DAIRY
 *1 small pot non-fat natural
  yoghurt*
 1 small pot whipping cream
SEAFOOD
 *350g (12oz) red snapper
  fillets*
GROCERY
 *1 small container stoned
  green olives (6 needed)*
 *1 small pack wholemeal rolls
  (2 needed)*
 1 miniature Pernod bottle
STAPLES
 Red wine vinegar
 Dijon mustard
 Olive oil
 Garlic
 Artificial sweetener
 Salt
 Black peppercorns

helpful hints

- Use toasted sesame oil if available in your local supermarket. It gives a smoky flavour.
- Chinese cabbage is also known as Chinese leaves. It has thin, crisp, pale green leaves. Any firm lettuce can be substituted.
- Hoisin sauce is a mixture of soya beans, garlic, chilli peppers and spices. It can be found in the Chinese section of the supermarket.
- Rice vinegar can be bought in the Asian section of the supermarket. Half a tablespoon of water mixed with ½ tablespoon distilled white vinegar may be used as a substitute.

countdown

- Prepare walnuts and chicken.
- While chicken marinates, prepare all other ingredients.
- Stir-fry Sweet and Sour Cabbage.
- Using same wok, stir-fry the chicken dish.

chicken and walnuts in lettuce puffs

The nutritional analysis for this recipes fits the Which Carbs phase.

Stir-fried chicken, walnuts and vegetables served in lettuce puffs is one of my favourite dishes in a Chinese restaurant. Hoisin sauce spooned over crisp, cool lettuce and then topped with warm chicken and vegetables creates a taste and texture sensation.

I asked the chef at a top Chinese restaurant why cooking in a wok at home doesn't produce the same results as when food is prepared in a restaurant. Here's his advice: don't overcrowd the wok. Cook small portions. Use a wok that is about 50cm (20in) in diameter; if using a smaller wok, use even smaller portions. Heat the wok until it is almost smoking, then add the oil. Drizzle the oil around the sides, swirling to coat the wok, and wait about 5 seconds before adding the other ingredients.

chicken and walnuts in lettuce puffs

110g (4oz) boneless, skinless chicken breasts, cut into 1cm (½ in) pieces
1 tablespoon bottled oyster sauce
2 tablespoons walnut pieces
3 teaspoons sesame oil
1 teaspoon crushed fresh ginger or ½ teaspoon ground ginger
1 medium garlic clove, crushed
40g (1½oz) diced carrots
50g (2oz) diced shiitake mushrooms
75g (3oz) sliced water chestnuts
½ tablespoon rice vinegar
50ml (2fl oz) hoisin sauce
8 small iceberg lettuce cups (inner leaves from lettuce that curve into a cup)

Place chicken in a bowl with the oyster sauce and leave to stand for 10 minutes. Heat wok over high heat and add walnut pieces. Toast in wok for 1–2 minutes or until slightly coloured. Remove and set aside. Heat wok over high heat. Add 1 teaspoon sesame oil. Add ginger and cook, stirring, until fragrant, about 10 seconds. Add chicken and oyster sauce and stir-fry for 1 minute. Add garlic, carrots, mushrooms and water chestnuts. Stir-fry for 2 minutes. Add remaining 2 teaspoons sesame oil and rice vinegar. Cook to heat through for a few seconds. Add walnuts and toss to coat. Remove from heat.

To serve: divide chicken, hoisin sauce and lettuce cups between 2 dinner plates. Spread a small spoonful of hoisin sauce on a lettuce cup, spoon in some of the chicken mixture, wrap in lettuce cup, and eat like a sandwich.
Makes 2 servings.

Per serving: 541 calories, 58.3 grams protein, 27.2 grams carbohydrate, 23.6 grams fat (3.6 saturated), 145 milligrams cholesterol, 797 milligrams sodium, 4.1 grams fibre

sweet and sour cabbage

Several drops hot pepper sauce
1 tablespoon hoisin sauce
2 tablespoons Chinese rice vinegar
Artificial sweetener equivalent to
*   2 teaspoons sugar*
½ teaspoon salt
1 teaspoon sesame oil
225g (8oz) Chinese cabbage,
*   thinly sliced*
1 medium red pepper, seeded and
*   sliced*

Mix together hot pepper sauce, hoisin sauce, Chinese rice vinegar, sweetener and salt. Heat wok to smoking and add sesame oil. When oil is smoking, add cabbage and red pepper. Stir-fry for 2 minutes. Pour in sauce. Toss well, spoon into a bowl, and leave to stand until chicken dish is ready. This can be served hot or cold. Do not wash the wok. It can be used for the chicken dish.

Makes 2 servings.

Per serving: 81 calories, 2.3 grams protein, 12.8 grams carbohydrate, 3.0 grams fat (0.4 saturated), 0 milligrams cholesterol, 691 milligrams sodium, 2.2 grams fibre

dessert

2 oranges

Slice oranges in quarters and place on 2 dessert plates.

Makes 2 servings.

Per serving: 62 calories, 1.2 grams protein, 15.4 grams carbohydrate, 0.2 grams fat (0 saturated), 0 milligrams cholesterol, 0 milligrams sodium, 3.1 grams fibre

shopping list

FRUIT AND VEG
*   1 small piece fresh ginger or*
*   ground ginger*
*   1 small packet shiitake*
*   mushrooms (50g/2oz*
*   needed)*
*   1 small head iceberg lettuce*
*   1 small head Chinese*
*   cabbage (Chinese leaves)*
*   1 medium red pepper*
*   2 oranges*
MEAT
*   110g (4oz) boneless, skinless*
*   chicken breasts*
GROCERY
*   1 small bottle oyster sauce*
*   1 small bottle sesame oil*
*   1 small bottle hoisin sauce*
*   1 small tin sliced water*
*   chestnuts*
*   1 small packet walnut pieces*
STAPLES
*   Carrots*
*   Garlic*
*   Rice vinegar*
*   Hot pepper sauce*
*   Artificial sweetener*
*   Salt*

steak in port wine

The nutritional analysis for this recipe fits the Which Carbs phase.

This typical French bistro dish is a delicious recipe and very simple to prepare. The shallots and mushrooms provide the base for the wine sauce.

Shallots have a milder flavour than onions. They are used in many sauces because their cellular structure allows them to melt into the sauce.

To flambé, if using gas, warm the cognac in the pan for a few seconds and then tip the pan so that the gas flame will ignite the liquid. Remove from the heat and wait for the flame to die down. If using an electric hob, throw a lighted match into the warmed cognac. When the flame dies down, remove the match. Keep a frying pan lid nearby for safety.

Brown rice takes about 45 minutes to cook. There are several brands of quick-cooking brown rice available. Their cooking time ranges from 10 to 30 minutes. I find the 30-minute rice has more flavour, but any quick-cooking rice will work for this dinner.

helpful hints

● *Beef fillet medallions or steaks may not be in the meat cabinet. Ask the butcher to cut two 175g (6oz) beef fillet medallions for you. Or buy a 350g (12oz) piece of beef fillet and cut it into 2 steaks at home.*

● *Haricots vert or small French green beans can be found in most supermarkets. They are pencil thin and take only a few minutes to cook. If unavailable, use fresh green beans and cut into 5cm (2in) pieces.*

● *To save washing another pan, use the same frying pan for beans and steak.*

● *Slice mushrooms and shallots in a food processor fitted with a thin slicing blade.*

countdown

● *Start rice.*
● *Make beans.*
● *Make steak.*

steak in port wine

1 teaspoon rapeseed oil
2 x 175g (6oz) beef fillet medallions
Salt and freshly ground black pepper
50ml (2fl oz) cognac
5 medium shallots, peeled and thinly sliced
110g (4oz) portobello mushrooms, thinly sliced
50ml (2fl oz) dry port wine
115ml (4fl oz) fat-free, low-sodium chicken stock
2 tablespoons single cream
2 tablespoons chopped parsley

Heat oil in a non-stick frying pan just large enough to hold the fillets in one layer over medium heat. Add the steaks and brown for 2 minutes, turn and brown 2 minutes more for a 2.5cm (1in) thick steak. Add salt and pepper to taste to the cooked sides. If steak is 5–7.5cm (2–3in) thick, lower the heat to medium and sauté the fillets 3 minutes for rare, 5–6 minutes for medium rare. Add the cognac to the steak and flambé. Remove steak to a plate and cover with another plate or foil to keep warm. Add the shallots to the pan and sauté until golden, about 2 minutes. Do not let them turn dark brown or black. Add the mushrooms and sauté for 3 minutes. Add the port. Raise the heat to high and reduce the sauce for 1 minute. Add the chicken stock and reduce the sauce by half, about 1 minute. Stir in cream, and spoon sauce over steaks. Sprinkle with parsley.
Makes 2 servings.

Per serving: 470 calories, 38.6 grams protein, 11.7 grams carbohydrate, 19.0 grams fat (7.1 saturated), 115 milligrams cholesterol, 247 milligrams sodium, 0 grams fibre

brown rice

*50g (2oz) 30-minute quick cooking
brown rice*
*Salt and freshly ground black
pepper to taste*

Bring a large saucepan with 2–3 litres (4–5pints)
of water to the boil. Add the rice and boil for 30
minutes or according to packet instructions.
Drain and add salt and pepper to taste. Divide
rice between 2 plates and place steak on top.
Spoon sauce over steak and rice.
Makes 2 servings.

Per serving: 85 calories, 2.5 grams protein, 17.5 grams
carbohydrate, 0.8 grams fat (0.2 saturated),
0 milligrams cholesterol, 0 milligrams sodium,
.0 gram fibre

french green beans

2 teaspoons rapeseed oil
1 medium garlic clove, unpeeled
*225g (8oz) haricots vert (French
green beans), trimmed*
*Salt and freshly ground black
pepper*

Heat oil in a non-stick frying pan on medium-
high heat. Add garlic and beans and sauté for 5
minutes or until beans are tender but firm.
Remove garlic clove and add salt and pepper
to taste.
Makes 2 servings.

Per serving: 88 calories, 2.5 grams protein, 10.3 grams
carbohydrate, 5.0 grams fat (0.6 saturated),
0 milligrams cholesterol, 4 milligrams sodium,
2.2 grams fibre

shopping list

FRUIT AND VEG
   5 medium shallots
   *110g (4oz) portobello
      mushrooms*
   *1 small bunch chopped
      parsley*
   *225g (8oz) haricots vert
      (French green beans)*
DAIRY
   1 small pot single cream
MEAT
   *2 x 175g (6oz) beef fillet
      medallions*
GROCERY
   1 small bottle dry port wine
   1 small bottle cognac
STAPLES
   Garlic
   *30-minute quick-cooking
      brown rice*
   Rapeseed oil
   *Fat-free, low-sodium chicken
      stock*
   Salt
   Black peppercorns

right carbs

weekend

meals

indian-spiced chicken

This fits the nutritional guidelines for the Right Carbs phase.

Tandoori chicken with its delicate blend of spices and intriguing aroma is cooked in a clay oven and heated by charcoal. All of the spices can be found in the supermarket.

indian-spiced chicken

350g (12oz) boneless, skinless
  chicken breasts
225ml (8fl oz) non-fat natural
  yoghurt, drained
15g (1/2oz) fresh mint leaves plus
  2 tablespoons, chopped
1cm (1/2in) fresh ginger, peeled
  and chopped
1 teaspoon ground coriander
Pinch cayenne
Artificial sweetener equivalent to
  2 teaspoons sugar
2 teaspoons rapeseed oil
225g (8oz) frozen chopped onion
2 medium garlic cloves, crushed
Salt and freshly ground black
  pepper

Remove fat from chicken and make 3 or 4 long slits in meat to allow marinade to penetrate. Mix yoghurt, 15g (1/2oz) chopped mint, ginger, coriander, cayenne and sweetener together. Divide in half and reserve half the marinade in a separate bowl. Add chicken to half the marinade and let marinate for 10 minutes. Turn once during this time. Heat oil in a non-stick frying pan just large enough to hold chicken in 1 layer over medium-high heat. Remove chicken from marinade and discard marinade. Add onion, garlic and chicken to the pan. Brown chicken for 3 minutes. Turn and brown for 2 minutes. Sprinkle salt and pepper to taste over cooked sides. Lower heat to medium. Spoon reserved marinade over chicken, cover, and cook for 5 minutes. A meat thermometer should read 70ºC/160ºF. Sprinkle with remaining 2 tablespoons mint and serve. *Makes 2 servings.*

> Per serving: 428 calories, 60.8 grams protein, 19.5 grams carbohydrate, 12.6 grams fat (2.5 saturated), 147 milligrams cholesterol, 223 milligrams sodium, 0 grams fibre

rice and spinach pilaf

1 teaspoon rapeseed oil
225g (8oz) frozen chopped onion
150g (5oz) spinach
75g (3oz) basmati rice
225ml (8fl oz) fat-free, low-sodium
  chicken stock
1/2 teaspoon ground cumin
Salt and freshly ground black
  pepper

Heat oil in a medium-sized non-stick frying pan on medium-high heat. Add onion and spinach. Sauté for 2 minutes. Add rice and sauté for 1 minute. Add chicken stock and cumin. When liquid comes to a simmer, lower heat to medium, cover, and simmer for 15 minutes. Remove from heat, add salt and pepper to taste and serve. *Makes 2 servings.*

> Per serving: 249 calories, 8.8 grams protein, 47.7 grams carbohydrate, 2.8 grams fat (0.4 saturated), 0 milligrams cholesterol, 368 milligrams sodium, 3.6 grams fibre

helpful hints

● Fresh coriander can be used instead of fresh mint. A quick way to chop mint is to snip the leaves off the stem with scissors.

countdown

● Marinate chicken.
● Start spinach and rice.
● Complete chicken.
● Complete rice.

shopping list

FRUIT AND VEG
  1 small piece fresh ginger
  1 bag washed, ready-to-eat
    spinach (150g/5oz
    needed)
  1 small bunch fresh mint
DAIRY
  1 small pot non-fat natural
    yoghurt
MEAT
  350g (12oz) boneless,
    skinless chicken breasts
GROCERY
  1 small jar ground coriander
  1 small packet basmati rice
STAPLES
  Garlic
  Rapeseed oil
  Fat-free, low-sodium chicken
    stock
  Artificial sweetener
  Ground cumin
  Frozen chopped onion
  Cayenne pepper
  Salt
  Black peppercorns

pan-seared tuna with mango salsa

The nutritional analysis for these recipes fits the Right Carbs phase.

Pan searing is a perfect way to cook fish. The outside becomes crisp while the inside remains tender and moist. Toasting cumin and coriander seeds in the frying pan allows their natural oils to be released for a more concentrated flavour.

Brown rice takes about 45 minutes to cook. There are several brands of quick-cooking brown rice available. Their cooking time ranges from 10 to 30 minutes. The 10-minute rice is needed for this recipe.

The Lemon Chiffon is made with jelly and needs to be made at least 2 hours in advance. For a quick dessert, serve 1 orange per person.

helpful hints

● Pan searing requires that the frying pan be very hot. Add the fish only when you see smoke rising from the pan.

● Use a non-stick frying pan that is just large enough to hold the tuna.

● Peaches or plums can be substituted for mango.

● To cube mango, slice off each side of the mango as close to the stone as possible. Take the mango half in your hand, skin side down. Score the fruit in a criss-cross pattern through to the skin. Bend the skin backwards so that the cubes pop up. Slice the cubes away from the skin. Score and slice any fruit left on the stone.

countdown

● Make dessert 2 hours ahead.
● Make Saffron Pilaf.
● Make salsa.
● Make tuna.

pan-seared tuna with mango salsa

Salsa
1 ripe mango, cut into cubes
   (about 225g/8oz)
2 tablespoons chopped red onion
1 teaspoon ground cumin
1 tablespoon balsamic vinegar
Several drops hot pepper sauce
15g (1/2oz) chopped fresh
   coriander
1 tablespoon cumin seeds
1 tablespoon coriander seeds
1 teaspoon olive oil
350g (12oz) tuna steak
Salt
2 wholemeal rolls

To prepare the salsa, combine mango, red onion, ground cumin, balsamic vinegar, hot pepper sauce and coriander in a bowl. Toss well. Taste for seasoning and add more cumin if needed.

To prepare the tuna, place cumin and coriander seeds in a medium non-stick frying pan over medium heat. Toss for 2 minutes and remove from heat. Place in a food processor or mini-processor and coarsely chop. Add olive oil and blend for a few seconds.

Rinse tuna and pat dry with kitchen paper. Spoon the spice mixture over both sides of the tuna, pressing the seeds into the fish with the back of the spoon. Heat the same frying pan on high. It needs to be smoking before the tuna is added. Brown tuna for 1 minute on one side and turn. Brown for another minute and lower heat to medium-high. Cook for another 3–4 minutes. Add a little salt to taste. Remove tuna to 2 plates, spoon salsa on top, and serve with rolls.
Makes 2 servings.

Per serving: 322 calories, 37.2 grams protein,
19.6 grams carbohydrate, 10.3 grams fat
(2.4 saturated), 59 milligrams cholesterol,
203 milligrams sodium, 1.1 grams fibre

saffron pilaf

1 teaspoon olive oil

175g (6oz) 10-minute quick-
cooking brown rice

225ml (8fl oz) water

⅛ teaspoon saffron

Salt and freshly ground black
pepper

Heat olive oil in a medium non-stick frying pan over medium heat. Add rice and sauté for 1 minute. Add water and saffron. Bring to a simmer and cover. Simmer for 15 minutes. Add salt and pepper to taste.

Makes 2 servings.

Per serving: 148 calories, 3.8 grams protein, 26.3 grams carbohydrate, 3.5 grams fat (0.5 saturated), 0 milligrams cholesterol, 0 milligrams sodium, 1.5 grams fibre

lemon chiffon

125g (4½oz) sugar-free low
calorie lemon jelly

110g (4oz) low-fat ricotta cheese

Make up jelly according to packet instructions, using 6 large ice cubes instead of cold water for a quick set. Leave to set for 1 hour. Whip with a whisk, and fold in the ricotta cheese. Spoon into 2 glass dessert bowls or dishes and leave to set for 1 hour.

Makes 2 servings.

Per serving: 174 calories, 3.6 grams protein, 19.3 grams carbohydrate, 1 gram fat (0.3 saturated), 0 milligrams cholesterol, 236 milligrams sodium, 0.6 grams fibre

shopping list

FRUIT AND VEG
  1 bunch fresh coriander
  1 ripe mango
DAIRY
  1 small pot low-fat ricotta
    cheese
SEAFOOD
  350g (12oz) tuna steak
GROCERY
  2 wholemeal rolls
  1 small jar cumin seeds
  1 small jar coriander seeds
  1 small packet saffron
    threads
  1 packet sugar-free, low
    calorie lemon jelly
STAPLES
  Red onion
  Hot pepper sauce
  Balsamic vinegar
  Ground cumin
  Olive oil
  10-minute quick-cooking
    brown rice
  Salt
  Black peppercorns

helpful hints

- *Look for unsweetened apple sauce with 100 calories, 30 grams sodium and 30 grams carbohydrates per 225ml (8fl oz).*
- *Standard pork chops can be used instead of boneless ones. Either cut the bone out before cooking or increase the cooking time for the chops by about 5 minutes.*
- *A quick way to chop chives is to snip them with scissors.*

countdown

- *Start lentils.*
- *Make pork chops and relish.*
- *Finish lentils.*
- *Make dessert.*

pork chops with apple relish

The nutritional analysis for this recipes fits the Right Carbs phase.

Sweet and tart apple relish garnishes a sautéed boneless pork chop for this quick weekend dinner. This recipe calls for a Gala apple. It's a sweet, moderately crisp, juicy apple that holds its shape well and adds just the right amount of sweetness to the relish. If you can't find Gala apples, use another type of your choice.

You can buy boneless, butterflied pork chops in the supermarket. They have very little fat and cook quickly.

Shallots have a milder flavour than onions. They are used in many sauces because their cellular structure allows them to melt into the sauce.

pork chops with apple relish

1 teaspoon rapeseed oil
2 x 175g (6oz) boneless loin pork chops
Salt and freshly ground black pepper
1 medium Gala apple, cored and coarsely chopped
1 medium shallot, chopped
2 tablespoons apple cider vinegar
Artificial sweetener equivalent to 2 teaspoons sugar

Heat rapeseed oil in a small non-stick frying pan over medium-high heat. Add pork chops and brown for 2 minutes. Turn and brown second side for 2 minutes. Season the cooked sides to taste with salt and pepper. Reduce heat to medium and cook for 4 minutes. A meat thermometer should read 70ºC/160ºF.

While pork chops cook, mix apple, shallot, apple cider vinegar and sweetener together in a small bowl. Add salt and pepper to taste.

Place pork chops on individual dinner plates and spoon apple relish on top.

Makes 2 servings.

Per serving: 325 calories, 45.5 grams protein, 12.7 grams carbohydrate, 10.1 grams fat (3.0 saturated), 146 milligrams cholesterol, 106 milligrams sodium, 1.9 grams fibre

toasted walnut lentils

225ml (8fl oz) fat-free, low-sodium chicken stock
225ml (8fl oz) water
110g (4oz) dried lentils
2 tablespoons walnut pieces
Salt and freshly ground black pepper
15g (½oz) snipped chives

Bring chicken stock and water to a rolling boil in a medium-sized saucepan over high heat. Slowly add lentils so that the water continues to boil. Reduce the heat to medium-low, cover with a lid and simmer for 20 minutes. Meanwhile place walnuts on a foil-lined baking tray and toast in a toaster oven or under a grill for several minutes. Watch them carefully. They burn easily. Remove lid and continue to cook lentils over high heat, until any remaining liquid has been absorbed. Season with salt and pepper to taste. Toss with walnuts and chives.
Makes 2 servings.

Per serving: 245 calories, 16.8 grams protein, 29.7 grams carbohydrate, 7.9 grams fat (0.7 saturated), 0 milligrams cholesterol, 285 milligrams sodium, 15.4 grams fibre

cranberry apple sauce

450ml (16fl oz) unsweetened apple sauce
2 tablespoons dried cranberries
50ml (2fl oz) water

Divide apple sauce between 2 dessert bowls. Microwave cranberries with water for 1 minute. Drain cranberries, divide in half and stir into the apple sauce.
Makes 2 servings.

Per serving: 145 calories, 0.4 grams protein, 42.1 grams carbohydrate, 0.2 grams fat (0.1 saturated), 0 milligrams cholesterol, 31 milligrams sodium, 4 grams fibre

shopping list

FRUIT AND VEG
  1 medium Gala apple
  1 medium shallot
  1 small bunch chives
MEAT
  2 x 175g (6oz) boneless loin pork chops
GROCERY
  1 small bottle apple cider vinegar
  1 small packet dried lentils
  1 small packet walnut pieces
  1 small jar unsweetened apple sauce
  1 small packet dried cranberries
STAPLES
  Rapeseed oil
  Fat-free, low-sodium chicken stock
  Artificial sweetener
  Salt
  Black peppercorns

entertaining

This section is geared to making parties that don't take all day to prepare. I love to have friends over, but find it hard to spend days shopping and cooking. I also want to serve food that's fun to eat and won't break the calorie bank. These parties let you splurge a little and still keep within the overall guidelines of the low-carbohydrate lifestyle.

They are designed for eight people to show you dishes you can make to follow a theme and create an atmosphere. The foods and quantities fit within the guidelines for the phase indicated at the top of each menu. You may want to make more and have some leftovers rather than run short (some guests may take more of a food they prefer and less of another).

Every detail of these parties has been planned for you including

- A shopping list with the amounts you will need
- A countdown for the days prior to and the day including the party

- The countdown indicates when to buy the ingredients, when to prepare each dish, and how to store and reheat or prepare them for serving.

Most of the recipes need very little preparation and many can be made ahead. There's almost no last-minute preparation.

Choose from the different party styles to best suit your occasion

- The Buffet for Friends is perfect for football or other sports-related parties, picnics or those times when you have a group over for a Sunday brunch after a family event.
- Prepare the Italian Supper for Friends for simple gatherings or casual Saturday nights. It is perfect for any season of the year.
- The Barbecue Party is easy to assemble, set up outside or in, and creates a fun atmosphere for your entertaining.
- It seems that a majority of guests want to hang out in the kitchen. So, serve the Casual Soup Supper right in the kitchen with the soup in a large pot on the

stove and the sandwiches and salad on the kitchen work surfaces.

- For the times you want an elegant dinner, the Dinner Party for Eight is your answer. Much of it can be made ahead and there are exact instructions for preparing the dishes so that you don't have to spend the evening in the kitchen.

Here are some general guidelines for drinks that will fit any of these parties:

- To keep within the low-carbohydrate guidelines, count 1 glass of alcohol or wine per person and choose from this list for some other interesting drinks for them to try.
- Make a jug of strong-flavoured coffee, such as hazelnut or amaretto, and cool in the refrigerator. Serve over ice in tall attractive glasses. Be sure to place ice in the jug just before serving or serve the ice in a bucket on the side.
- Stay away from flavoured syrups for coffee. They usually are made with a sugar syrup base.
- Make a jug of flavoured iced tea such as peach, berry or apple cinnamon. Or make a mixture of peach and apple cinnamon tea together. Set out glasses with a slice of the particular type of fruit in each glass.
- Serve no-sugar-added, flavoured sparkling water with a twist of lemon or lime.
- Serve unusual-flavoured diet soft drinks.

Decorate your table for the occasion. Let your table set the atmosphere and create a warm, welcoming feeling. A TV lifestyle expert gave me some tips on how to make your buffet table look attractive.

Decorate around the theme of the meal by using

- Italian pottery and colours for an Italian meal
- The colours of the teams playing for a sports party
- Colours from your garden flowers for an outdoor or barbecue party
- A tone-on-tone theme (for example, different shades of white and cream) for an elegant party.

Fill the buffet table with enticing objects. Take your coloured napkins and go around the house looking for objects that go with them. Gather them together and see what looks best on the table. These can be pottery, vases, candlesticks, garden baskets, flowerpots, an old child's toy or a miniature wooden wheelbarrow. Select pieces that go with your theme or colours and set them on the table. Remove those that don't look right until you have an attractive display. Use these objects as bases for flower arrangements, napkin and cutlery holders, or just as a design element on the table. This will make your table fun and inviting without having to spend hours preparing a groaning display of food.

italian supper
for friends

italian supper for friends

This party fits the guidelines for the Which Carbs section.

This Italian meal is perfect for a casual buffet. Most of the recipes can be made ahead, leaving just a few things to do on the day.

Menu

Garden Crudités and Dips

Chicken Tonnato

Lentil and Rice Salad

String Beans with Crumbled Gorgonzola

White Chocolate Whip

Countdown

Two days ahead

● Shop for ingredients.

Morning of the party

● Make dessert, place in dessert glasses or dishes, and refrigerate.

● Slice fennel, arrange crudités platter, wrap and refrigerate. Make dip.

● Arrange string beans on a platter, wrap and refrigerate.

● Arrange chicken on platter with sauce, peppers, capers and olives. Wrap and refrigerate.

One hour before guests arrive

● Remove finished dishes from refrigerator to bring to room temperature.

● Drizzle dressing on green beans and sprinkle cheese on top.

One day ahead

● Poach chicken and make sauce.

● Cut courgette for crudités, and store in plastic bags in the refrigerator.

● Make Lentil and Rice Salad and place in attractive bowl. Wrap and refrigerate.

● Blanch green beans, place in plastic bag, and refrigerate.

shopping list

Buy 2 days ahead of party

FRUIT AND VEG
  225g (8oz) broccoli florets
  675g (1½lb) haricots vert
  1 small courgette
  2 medium fennel bulbs
DAIRY
  1 large pot non-fat natural
    yoghurt
  825g (30oz) low-fat ricotta
    cheese
  1 packet crumbled
    Gorgonzola
MEAT
  8 x 175g (6oz) boneless,
    skinless chicken breasts
GROCERY
  1 small jar honey
  1 small packet dried lentils
  1 small packet basmati rice
  1 small container saffron
    threads
  1 packet pinenuts
  1 small jar ground coriander
  1 small bottle dry white wine
  1 small tin anchovy fillets
  1 jar sweet peppers

1 jar capers
1 container stoned black
  olives (18 needed)
2 packets instant fat-free,
  sugar-free, white
  chocolate pudding mix
  (75g/3oz needed)
1 small packet semi-sweet
  chocolate
STAPLES
Staples
Olive oil spray
Red onions
Garlic
Dijon mustard
Fat-free, low-sodium chicken
  stock
Reduced-fat mayonnaise
Olive oil and vinegar dressing
Olive oil
Salt
Black peppercorns
Tinned tuna packed in water

garden crudités

225g (8oz) broccoli florets,
   washed and cut in half, if large
1 small courgette, washed and
   sliced diagonally in 0.5cm (¹/₂in)
   slices
2 medium bulbs fennel, sliced
115ml (4fl oz) non-fat natural
   yoghurt
2 tablespoons honey
2 tablespoons Dijon mustard

Arrange the vegetables on a platter or plate. Mix yoghurt, honey and mustard together and place in a small bowl. Or slice the top off a small red cabbage and hollow out the inside. Spoon the dressing into the cabbage and serve near the crudités. Makes 8 servings.

Per serving: 56 calories, 2.2 grams protein, 9.1 grams carbohydrate, 0.4 grams fat (0 saturated), 0 milligrams cholesterol, 110 milligrams sodium, 0.8 grams fibre

helpful hints

● If you can find one, use a yellow courgette for extra colour.
● Any type of pre-cut vegetables can be added.
● Use cut vegetables from the salad bar. Pick and choose the vegetables that are in season.
● To slice fennel, cut off stem and leaves and slice the bulb only.

chicken tonnato

This is a traditional summer Italian dish that is perfect for buffets. The secret to keeping the chicken moist is to gently poach it and let it cool in the poaching liquid.

8 x 175g (6oz) boneless, skinless chicken breasts

115ml (4fl oz) dry white wine

225ml (8fl oz) fat-free, low-sodium chicken stock

Salt and freshly ground black pepper

6 anchovy fillets

250g (9oz) tinned tuna, packed in water

150ml (5fl oz) reduced-fat mayonnaise

150ml (5fl oz) non-fat natural yoghurt

1½ teaspoons lemon juice

2 large peppers, thinly sliced

6 tablespoons capers, drained and rinsed

18 stoned black olives, halved

Remove fat from chicken. Add wine and chicken stock to a large saucepan. Bring to the boil on medium-high heat. Add chicken and then enough warm water to make sure all of the chicken is covered by liquid. Bring to a simmer, lower heat to medium-low and gently simmer, uncovered, for 5 minutes. Do not boil the chicken. Remove from heat and let chicken cool in the liquid for 15 minutes (reserve 115ml/ 4fl oz of the poaching liquid). Sprinkle chicken with salt and pepper to taste.

While chicken cools, make the sauce. Rinse anchovy fillets and place in the bowl of a food processor with tuna, mayonnaise and yoghurt. Process until smooth. Add poaching liquid and continue to process. Add lemon juice and process to blend into sauce.

To serve, remove chicken from liquid and place on serving platter. Spoon enough sauce over chicken to coat. Serve remaining sauce on the side. Lay pimiento strips across chicken. Sprinkle capers over chicken and arrange the olives attractively. Cover and refrigerate until needed. Bring to room temperature before serving.

Per serving: 412 calories, 59.9 grams protein, 6.8 grams carbohydrate, 17.2 grams fat (3.4 saturated), 153 milligrams cholesterol, 1057 milligrams sodium, 0.7 grams fibre

lentil and rice salad

450ml (16fl oz) fat-free, low-
  sodium chicken stock
450ml (16fl oz) water
225g (8oz) lentils, rinsed to
  remove stones
110g (4oz) basmati rice, rinsed
½ teaspoon saffron threads
Salt and freshly ground black
  pepper
50g (2oz) pinenuts
350g (12oz) sliced red onion
6 garlic cloves, crushed
½ teaspoon ground coriander
2 tablespoons plus 2 teaspoons
  olive oil

Bring chicken stock and 225ml (8fl oz) water to the boil in a non-stick pan on medium-high heat. Add the lentils slowly so that the stock continues to boil. Lower heat to medium. Cover with a lid and simmer for 5 minutes. Add rice, saffron and remaining water to the lentils. Bring back to a simmer, cover, and simmer for 15 minutes. The liquid will be absorbed and the lentils cooked through, but firm. Add salt and pepper to taste. While lentils and rice cook, heat a non-stick frying pan on medium-high heat and add the pinenuts. Sauté pinenuts for 1–2 minutes or until golden. Be careful because the nuts burn easily. Remove and set aside. Heat 2 teaspoons olive oil in the same pan and add the onion. Sauté, without browning, for 5 minutes. Add the garlic and continue to sauté for another 5 minutes.

Place lentils, rice and onion in a large bowl and add the remaining 2 tablespoons oil, coriander and salt and pepper to taste. Toss well. Taste for seasoning and add more salt and pepper, if needed. Sprinkle toasted pinenuts on top and serve.

Makes 8 servings.

Per serving: 231 calories, 9.2 grams protein, 29.6 grams carbohydrate, 5.1 grams fat (0.7 saturated), 0 milligrams cholesterol, 144 milligrams sodium, 7.3 grams fibre

helpful hints

● Turmeric can be substituted for the saffron.

helpful hints

● A quick way to trim beans is to line them up with the ends together and slice off the tips. Turn bunch around to opposite ends, line them up, and slice off the tips.

● Large green beans can be used. Cut them into 10cm (4in) lengths before blanching.

● Any type of blue veined cheese can be used.

string beans with crumbled gorgonzola

675g (1³/₄lb) haricots vert (small green beans)

3 tablespoons olive oil and vinegar dressing

Salt and freshly ground black pepper

110g (4oz) crumbled Gorgonzola

Bring a medium-sized saucepan of water to the boil. Trim beans and add to boiling water. As soon as the water comes back to the boil, drain and plunge beans into a bowl of iced water. Drain. Place on platter, drizzle dressing over the top and toss. Add salt and pepper to taste. Sprinkle cheese on top.

Makes 8 servings.

Per serving: 64 calories, 3.5 grams protein, 5.1 grams carbohydrate, 3.6 grams fat (2.1 saturated), 10 milligrams cholesterol, 194 milligrams sodium, 1.1 grams fibre

white chocolate whip

825g (30oz) low-fat ricotta cheese

450ml (16fl oz) water

75g (3oz) fat-free, sugar-free instant white chocolate pudding powder

4 teaspoons grated semi-sweet chocolate

Whisk ricotta cheese and water together until smooth. This can be done in a food processor. Add the white chocolate pudding powder and whisk until smooth. Divide between 8 dessert bowls. Sprinkle ½ teaspoon grated chocolate on top of each dish.

Makes 8 servings.

Per serving: 114 calories, 0.1 grams protein, 4.9 grams carbohydrate, 0.2 grams fat (0.1 saturated), 0 milligrams cholesterol, 272 milligrams sodium, 0 grams fibre

dinner party
for eight

dinner party for eight

This dinner party fits the nutritional guidelines for the Which Carbs phase.

No need to spend all day making an elegant dinner party. These recipes are easy to make and you and your guests can enjoy the evening without worrying about the calories and carbs.

Menu

Bruschetta

Guinea Fowl in Red Wine

Brown Rice with Toasted Pinenuts

Roasted Asparagus with Red Pepper

Radicchio, Chicory and Watercress Salad

Berry Cups with Almond Sauce

Countdown

Two days ahead

- *Shop for ingredients.*

One day ahead

- *Make Guinea Fowl in Red Wine. Place in ovenproof casserole or dish in their sauce. Cover and refrigerate.*
- *Make Brown Rice with Toasted Pinenuts. Place in an oven-to-table dish, cover and refrigerate.*
- *Make Almond Sauce for dessert. Cover and refrigerate.*

Morning of the party

- *Assemble berry cups without sauce and wrap and refrigerate.*
- *Prepare asparagus ready for the oven. Cut off the woody ends, place on baking trays, roll in olive oil, and place in refrigerator.*
- *Wash watercress, radicchio and chicory; dry and place in salad bowl. Cover with clingfilm and refrigerate.*
- *Make bruschetta topping and refrigerate.*

One hour before guests arrive

- *Remove guinea fowl, rice, asparagus, berries and sauce from refrigerator.*

Thirty minutes before guests arrive

- *Pre-heat oven to 150ºC/300ºF/gas mark 2.*
- *Place guinea fowl in their sauce and rice in oven for 30 minutes to warm through.*
- *Remove salad from refrigerator and toss with dressing.*
- *Spoon topping for bruschetta on toasts and arrange on serving tray.*

Before dessert

- *Spoon sauce over berries just before serving.*

shopping list

Buy 2 days ahead of party

FRUIT AND VEG
1 medium tomato
1 medium head radicchio
2 medium heads chicory
1 bunch watercress
900g (2lb) asparagus
350g (12oz) button
    mushrooms
1 packet broccoli florets
    (275g/10oz needed)
Mixture of raspberries,
    strawberries and
    blueberries (1.1kg/2½lb
    berries needed)
DAIRY
1 pot reduced-fat crème
    fraiche (225ml/8fl oz
    needed)
MEAT
4 guinea fowl, about 900g
    (2lb) each
GROCERY
1 jar sweet peppers
    (450g/16oz needed)
1 packet flaked almonds
1 packet pinenuts

1 bottle almond essence
1 bottle red wine (Beaujolais
    or Burgundy)
STAPLES
30-minute quick-cooking
    brown rice
Olive oil spray
Red onion
Yellow onion
Carrots
Garlic
Wholemeal bread
Fat-free, low-sodium chicken
    stock
Olive oil
Balsamic vinegar
Olive oil and vinegar dressing
Artificial sweetener
Salt
Black peppercorns

bruschetta

Olive oil spray
225g (8oz) sliced red onion
2 garlic cloves, crushed
1 medium tomato, diced
½ tablespoon olive oil
1 teaspoon balsamic vinegar
Salt and freshly ground black
*   pepper*
4 slices of wholemeal toast, cut
*   into squares*

Heat a non-stick frying pan on medium-high heat. Spray with olive oil spray and add onion and garlic. Sauté for 10 minutes. The onion should be golden. Remove from heat and toss with tomatoes. Add olive oil, balsamic vinegar and salt and pepper to taste. Place in a bowl and refrigerate until needed.

To serve, spoon tomato mixture on to toast and place on serving platter.

Per serving: 56 calories, 1.6 grams protein, 7.9 grams carbohydrate, 1.9 grams fat (0.4 saturated), 0 milligrams cholesterol, 39 milligrams sodium, 0.5 grams fibre

helpful hints

● *Chicory should not be placed in water to clean. The leaves will turn brown. Just remove any damaged outer leaves and then wipe with damp kitchen paper.*

radicchio, chicory and watercress salad

1 medium head radicchio
1 bunch watercress
2 medium heads chicory
5 tablespoons olive oil and vinegar
*   dressing*

Wash radicchio and watercress and dry. Cut about 2.5cm (1in) off flat end of chicory and remove any torn or brown outer leaves. Wipe chicory with damp kitchen paper. Tear radicchio leaves into bite-sized pieces. Break large stems off watercress. Slice chicory into 2.5cm (1in) circles. When salad is dry, place in a salad bowl, cover with clingfilm, and refrigerate. Just before serving, toss with the dressing.

Makes 8 servings.

Per serving: 56 calories, 0.7 grams protein, 1.9 grams carbohydrate, 5.4 grams fat (1.9 saturated), 0 milligrams cholesterol, 59 milligrams sodium, 0.2 grams fibre

guinea fowl in red wine

4 guinea fowl, about 900g (2lb) each

Olive oil spray

450g (16oz) diced yellow onion

2 medium carrots, diced

4 medium garlic cloves, crushed

300ml (12fl oz) red wine (Beaujolais or Burgundy)

300ml (12fl oz) fat-free, low-sodium chicken stock

350g (12oz) sliced button mushrooms

Salt and freshly ground black pepper

Remove the fat from the cavity of the guinea fowl and split them in half. Heat 2 large non-stick frying pans just large enough to hold the halves in 1 layer over medium-high heat. Spray with olive oil spray. Brown the birds on both sides, about 5 minutes. Remove to a plate and pour off any excess fat. Add the diced onion, carrots and garlic to the pan. Sauté until the vegetables start to shrivel, about 5 minutes. Return guinea fowl halves to the pan, lower the heat to medium, and cover with a lid. Leave to cook until the guinea fowl are cooked through, about 20 minutes. A meat thermometer should read 80ºC/170ºF for white meat and 85ºC/180ºF for dark meat. Remove birds to a dish and cover with foil to keep warm. Pour off any remaining fat, add wine, and scrape the brown bits from the bottom of the pan while the wine simmers for about 2 minutes. Add the chicken stock and mushrooms. Simmer for 2 more minutes. Remove skin from guinea fowl and add salt and pepper to taste. If serving immediately, return the birds to the pan and let cook to warm through. Or place in an ovenproof serving platter and spoon sauce and vegetables on top. Cover and refrigerate. Remove from refrigerator and allow to come to room temperature, about 30 minutes. Place, covered with foil or a lid, in a 150ºC/300ºF/gas mark 2 oven for 20–30 minutes or until warmed through.

Makes 8 servings.

Per serving: 260 calories, 35.2 grams protein, 7.0 grams carbohydrate, 6.3 grams fat (1.6 saturated), 153 milligrams cholesterol, 215 milligrams sodium, 0.2 grams fibre

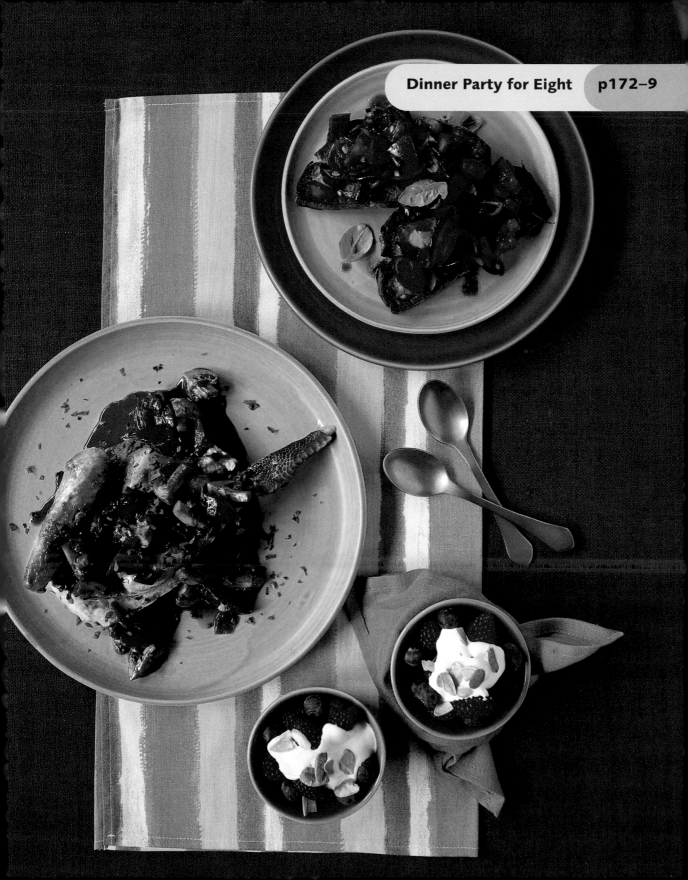

Dinner Party for Eight   **p172–9**

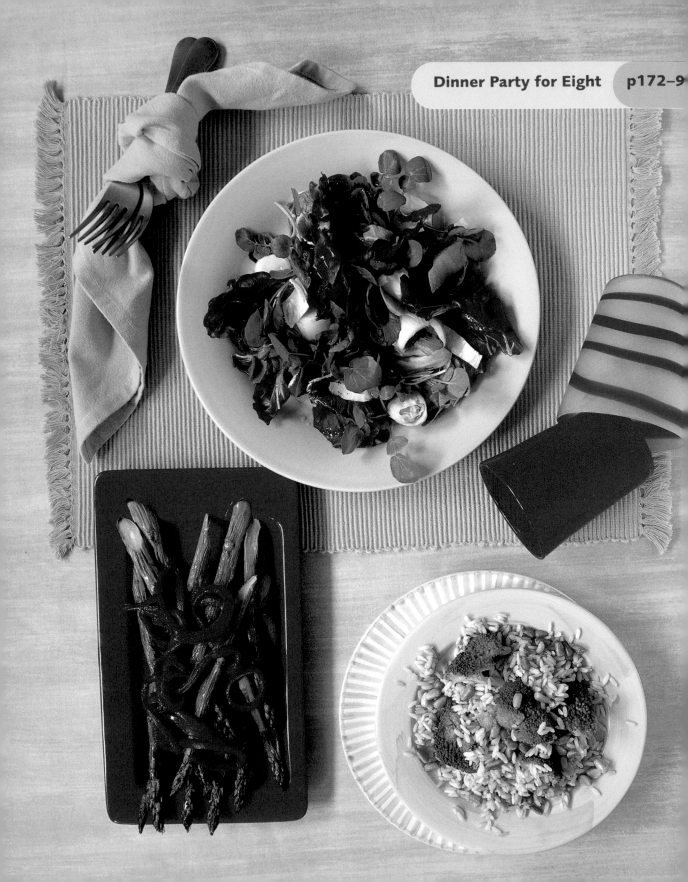

brown rice with toasted pinenuts

1 cup 30-minute quick-cooking brown rice
275g (10oz) broccoli florets
3 tablespoons pinenuts
1 tablespoon olive oil
Salt and freshly ground black pepper

Fill a large saucepan with 2–3 litres (4–5 pints) cold water. Add rice, cover with a lid and bring to a boil over high heat. When water comes to the boil, remove the lid, lower heat to medium-low and boil for 25 minutes. Add broccoli and continue to boil for 5 minutes. While rice boils, place pinenuts on a foil-lined baking tray and toast under a grill for 2–3 minutes or until golden. Be careful because the pinenuts burn easily.

When rice is cooked through, drain and toss with oil and salt and pepper to taste. Place in a serving bowl and sprinkle pinenuts on top.

Recipe may be made ahead until this point. Place rice in oven-to-tableware dish and store in the refrigerator. Before serving, bring to room temperature and place in pre-heated oven with guinea fowl for 30 minutes. Remove from oven and serve.

Makes 8 servings.

Per serving: 104 calories, 3.2 grams protein, 15.5 grams carbohydrate, 2.6 grams fat (0.4 saturated), 0 milligrams cholesterol, 10 milligrams sodium, 1.4 grams fibre

roasted asparagus with red peppers

¹/₂ *tablespoon olive oil*
Salt and freshly ground black pepper
900g (2lb) asparagus
450g (16oz) peppers

Pre-heat oven to 200ºC/400ºF/gas mark 6. Line a baking tray with foil and spoon oil on to foil. Add salt and pepper to taste. Add asparagus and roll in oil, making sure all spears are coated with oil and salt and pepper. Spread asparagus out to form 1 layer and roast in oven for 5 minutes. Remove asparagus and turn. Roast 10 more minutes for thick spears, 5 more minutes for thin ones. Remove from oven and arrange spears in straight rows on an oval serving platter. Cut peppers into thin strips and sprinkle over top.

Makes 8 servings.

Per serving: 33 calories, 2.0 grams protein, 5.0 grams carbohydrate, 1.1 grams fat
(0.2 saturated), 0 milligrams cholesterol, 8 milligrams sodium, 2.4 grams fibre

berry cups with almond sauce

1.1kg (2¹/₂lb) berries (mixture of raspberries, blueberries and strawberries)

2 teaspoons almond essence

Artificial sweetener equivalent to 2 teaspoons sugar

225ml (8fl oz) reduced-fat crème fraiche

3 tablespoons flaked almonds

Place berries in 8 small ramekins. Mix almond essence and sweetener into crème fraiche and spoon or dollop sauce on top of each one. Sauté almonds in a frying pan until just turning golden. Be careful toasting the almonds as they burn easily. Sprinkle almonds on top of sauce.
Makes 8 servings.

Per serving: 134 calories, 3 grams protein, 17.3 grams carbohydrate, 6.8 grams fat (2.7 saturated), 15 milligrams cholesterol, 20 milligrams sodium, 6.3 grams fibre

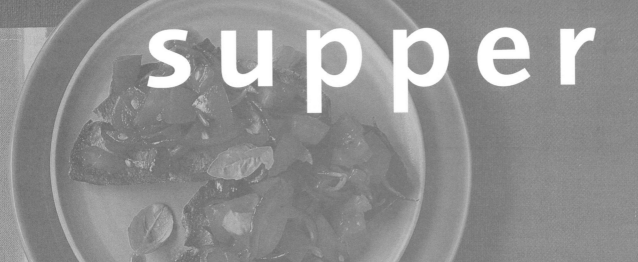

casual soup supper

casual soup supper

This meal fits the nutritional guidelines for the Right Carbs phase.

Whenever we have friends over, it seems that everyone ends up standing around the kitchen. I planned this party so that the kitchen is part of the fun. I make the soup and leave it in a large, colourful saucepan on the stove with a ladle in the soup. The bowls are nearby and people can help themselves. The sandwiches and salad are placed on the work surface. Everyone can help themselves on their way to finding a seat at the table.

Menu

Creamy Wild Mushroom Soup

Grilled Halibut Sandwich

Three Bean Salad

Mango Fool

Countdown

Two days ahead

● *Shop for most ingredients except the fish.*

One day ahead

● *Make soup, cover and refrigerate.*

Morning of the party

● *Buy fish.*

● *Make Mango Fool, place in attractive glass, and refrigerate.*

● *Make salad. Place in serving bowl. Cover and refrigerate.*

One hour ahead

● *Prepare ingredients for halibut sandwich.*

● *Remove salad from refrigerator.*

● *Remove soup from refrigerator.*

Fifteen minutes before guests arrive

● *Marinate fish.*

When guests arrive

● *Place soup on stove and heat. When soup is hot, lower heat to extra low and leave until served.*

● *Make halibut sandwich just before serving.*

● *Remove dessert from refrigerator.*

● *Spoon sauce over berries just before serving.*

shopping list

Buy 2 days ahead of party
except seafood

FRUIT AND VEG
  1 bunch fresh dill
  1 bunch spring onions
    (6 needed)
  350g (12oz) sliced
    portobello mushrooms
  2 medium tomatoes
  1 medium Spanish onion
  225g (8oz) green beans
  225g (8oz) yellow beans
  2 medium ripe mangoes
    (450g/1lb)
  1 bunch fresh mint
DAIRY
  1 small pot double cream
    (115ml/4fl oz needed)
  4 pots non-fat, sugar-free
    mango or tropical fruit
    yoghurt (900ml/32fl oz
    needed)
GROCERY
  1 small packet dried cèpes
    (mushrooms)
SEAFOOD
  8 X 175g (6oz) halibut fillets
    (purchase on the day of
    the party)

STAPLES:
  Red kidney beans (500g/
    18oz needed)
  Yellow onion
  Olive oil spray
  Balsamic vinegar
  Olive oil and vinegar dressing
  Flour
  Grated nutmeg
  Multi-grain bread
  Fat-free, low-sodium chicken
    stock
  Mayonnaise
  Lemons
  Salt
  Black peppercorns

creamy wild mushroom soup

Many 'wild' mushrooms are cultivated and don't have a strong flavour of the woods. Dried cèpes (called porcini in Italy) that have been gathered in the woods add a depth of flavour to this soup.

The secret to this soup is cooking the onion until it is sweet. Grated nutmeg gives the soup an intriguing flavour.

40g (1¹/₂oz) dried cèpe mushrooms

1.2 litres (40fl oz) hot water

Olive oil spray

1 large yellow onion, sliced

350g (12oz) sliced portobello mushrooms

1 tablespoon flour

900ml (32fl oz) fat-free, low-sodium chicken stock

8 tablespoons double cream

¹/₄ teaspoon grated nutmeg

Salt and freshly ground black pepper

Add dried cèpes to 225ml (8fl oz) hot water and leave to stand for 5 minutes. Drain, reserving the liquid, and slice. Strain liquid 2 to 3 times to remove sand.

Heat a large saucepan over medium-high heat and spray with olive oil spray. Add the onion and sauté for 2 minutes. Reduce heat to medium and continue to cook onion until golden, about 5 minutes. Do not brown onion. Add the portobello mushrooms and sauté for 2 minutes, stirring 1 or 2 times. Sprinkle flour on top and stir until absorbed, about 1 minute. Add chicken stock and remaining water. Lift reconstituted mushrooms from the hot water with a slotted spoon and add to the soup. Place a piece of kitchen towel in a sieve and strain the mushroom liquid into the soup. Bring to a boil. Simmer for 10 minutes. Add nutmeg and salt and pepper to taste.

Remove 225ml (8fl oz) soup to a blender or food processor and purée. Return to the soup. Spoon cream into soup and mix well. Taste for seasoning, adding more if necessary.

Makes 8 servings.

Per serving: 102 calories, 2.9 grams protein, 5.4 grams carbohydrate, 7.4 grams fat (3.8 saturated), 21 milligrams cholesterol, 288 milligrams sodium, 0 grams fibre

helpful hints

● *Slice onion and mushrooms in a food processor fitted with a 0.5cm (¹/₄in) slicing blade.*

● *Cook the onion until it is transparent, but not brown, to give the soup a sweet flavour.*

● *Morel mushrooms can be substituted.*

● *The soup can be made a day in advance. It will thicken on standing. Stir in a little stock when reheating.*

grilled halibut sandwich

Grilling fish gives great flavour. Grill on a barbecue, use your kitchen grill or simply sauté the fish in a frying pan. A renowned fish chef once showed me this method for grilling fish in advance. Sear the fish on the grill about 1 hour before needed and then place in a 140ºC/275ºF/gas mark 1 oven to finish cooking for about 30 minutes. For a 2.5cm (1in) thick fillet, sear 2 minutes per side and then place in oven.

helpful hints

- *Ask for the skin to be removed when you buy the fish.*
- *A quick way to chop dill is to snip the leaves with scissors.*
- *Make sure the grill bars are clean and spray them with vegetable cooking spray before grilling the fish.*

Any type of firm, white, non-oily fish fillet can be used.

8 x 175g (6oz) halibut fillets
450ml (16fl oz) balsamic vinegar
115ml (4fl oz) mayonnaise
2 tablespoons lemon juice
75g (3oz) snipped fresh dill
Salt and freshly ground black
    pepper
16 slices multi-grain bread
8 slices Spanish onion
8 slices tomato

Pre-heat grill. Rinse fish fillets and pat dry with kitchen paper. Place in a self-seal plastic bag and add balsamic vinegar. Marinate for 15 minutes. Meanwhile, mix mayonnaise with lemon juice and fold in 50g (2oz) dill, reserving the rest for garnish. Add salt and pepper to taste.

Remove fish from bag and pat dry with kitchen paper. Place on a barbecue grill 10cm (4in) from heat or under pre-heated kitchen grill. Grill for 2 minutes per side. Season cooked sides. While fish is cooking, toast the bread.

To serve, spread each slice of toast with a layer of mayonnaise. Place a fish fillet on each slice. Place onion slices on the fish and finish with tomato slices. Sprinkle with reserved dill. Serve as open sandwiches.

Makes 8 servings.

Per serving: 455 calories, 36.8 grams protein, 38.9 grams carbohydrate, 14.7 grams fat (2.5 saturated), 62 milligrams cholesterol, 570 milligrams sodium, 1.2 grams fibre

three bean salad

225g (8oz) green beans, trimmed
   and cut into 2.5cm (1in) pieces
225g (8oz) yellow beans, trimmed
   and cut into 2.5cm (1in) pieces
500g (18oz) cooked red kidney
   beans, rinsed and drained
6 spring onions, sliced
6 tablespoons olive oil and vinegar
   dressing
Salt and freshly ground black
   pepper

Bring a large saucepan filled with water to the boil. Add the green and yellow beans. As soon as the water returns to the boil, drain and refresh under ice cold water. Place in a large serving bowl and add the kidney beans, spring onions and dressing. Toss well. Add salt and pepper to taste. Toss once more.
Makes 8 servings.

Per serving: 141 calories, 4.4 grams protein, 17.1 grams carbohydrate, 6.7 grams fat (1.0 saturated), 0 milligrams cholesterol, 61 milligrams sodium, 2.2 grams fibre

mango fool

I was introduced to luscious, creamy fruit fools when I first moved to England. They are rich puddings, often made with tart green gooseberries. I have adapted this idea using fresh mangos and yoghurt.

225g (8oz) green beans, trimmed
   and cut into 2.5cm (1in) pieces
225g (8oz) yellow beans, trimmed
   and cut into 2.5cm (1in) pieces
500g (18oz) cooked red kidney
   beans, rinsed and drained
6 spring onions, sliced
6 tablespoons olive oil and vinegar
   dressing
Salt and freshly ground black
   pepper

Fold the mango cubes into the yoghurt and spoon into 8 attractive martini glasses or dessert bowls. Arrange a mint sprig in each glass. Refrigerate until 15 minutes before needed. Let come to room temperature before serving.
Makes 8 servings.

Per serving: 104 calories, 5.8 grams protein, 20.3 grams carbohydrate, 0.2 grams fat (0 saturated), 3 milligrams cholesterol, 96 milligrams sodium, 0.6 grams fibre

helpful hints

● *To blanch the beans and set their colour, they need to be plunged into iced water after they are drained. Fill a roasting tin with water and ice cubes and place near the sink. As soon as the beans are drained, plunge them into the iced water. When they are cold, drain.*

● *To cube a mango, slice off each side as close to the stone as possible. Cut a 2.5cm (1in) piece from one half. Remove the skin from the slice and cut into thin strips for a garnish. Take the mango half in your hand, skin side down. Score the fruit in a criss-cross pattern through to the skin. Bend the skin backwards so that the cubes pop up. Slice the cubes away from the skin. Repeat with the other half. Score and slice any fruit left on the stone.*

buffet for **friends**

buffet for friends

This meal fits the nutritional guidelines for the Right Carbs phase.

Informal family gatherings, brunch with friends, or 'open-house' parties all call for grazing foods that, when placed on a table, invite everyone to help themselves. This party needs very little attention during the festivities, leaving you to join in the fun.

Menu

Prawns in Lime-Mustard Sauce
Roasted Meat Platter with Horseradish and Honey Mustard Dressing
Tomato Platter
Pasta Salad
Frozen Yoghurt Berry Cup

Countdown

Two days ahead

● *Shop for ingredients.*

One day ahead

● *Arrange meat platter, wrap and refrigerate.*
● *Make sauces for meats. Cover and refrigerate.*
● *Make sauce for prawns.*
● *Poach prawns. Cover and refrigerate.*

Morning of the party

● *Arrange prawns on serving platter, wrap and refrigerate.*
● *Measure frozen yoghurt and place in dessert bowls. Place in freezer. Sprinkle berries around yoghurt just before serving.*
● *Slice tomatoes and assemble tomato platter.*
● *Make pasta salad.*

One hour before guests arrive

● *Remove prawns, meat and sauces from refrigerator and set on buffet table. Place prawn sauce near prawns and meat sauces near meat platter. Drizzle tomatoes with Honey Mustard Dressing. Place bread for meat platter in basket.*
● *Remove yoghurt bowls from freezer and sprinkle with berries 15 minutes before serving dessert.*

shopping list

Buy 2 days ahead of party

FRUIT AND VEG

2 limes

½ head red-leaf lettuce

1 bunch chives

1 bunch watercress

2 large red tomatoes

2 large yellow tomatoes

2 lemons

1 bunch dill

150g (5oz) broccoli florets

1 medium cucumber

2 medium red peppers

1.1kg (2½lb) fresh raspberries

DAIRY

1 pot non-fat natural yoghurt
(275ml/10fl oz needed)

DELI

350g (12oz) sliced lean deli
roast beef

350g (12oz) sliced roast
turkey breast

350g (12oz) lean sliced ham
(no honey-baked or glazed)

SEAFOOD

675g (1¾lb) prawns, peeled
and deveined

GROCERY

1 bottle horseradish

1 jar honey-flavoured mustard

225g (8oz) wholemeal penne
or other wholemeal short-
cut pasta

1 carton low-fat, frozen
strawberry yoghurt
(900ml/32fl oz needed)

2 packets thin-sliced rye bread
(32 slices needed)

STAPLES

Mayonnaise

Dijon mustard

Reduced-fat mayonnaise

Salt

Black peppercorns

prawns in lime-mustard sauce

675g (1³/₄lb) prawns, cooked, peeled and deveined
6 tablespoons mayonnaise
2 teaspoons Dijon mustard
1¹/₂ tablespoons lime juice

Arrange prawns in a circle, tails pointed out, on a serving platter. Mix mayonnaise, mustard and lime juice together in a small bowl. Place the bowl in the centre of the platter.
Makes 8 servings.

Per serving: 148 calories, 3.8 grams protein, 26.3 grams carbohydrate, 3.5 grams fat (0.5 saturated), 0 milligrams cholesterol, 0 milligrams sodium, 1.5 grams fibre

helpful hints

● *Shelled prawns are available at most supermarket seafood counters. The slightly higher cost is worth the time saved.*
● *If you're pressed for time, buy ready-cooked prawns from the seafood department of the supermarket.*
● *You can substitute lemon juice for the lime juice*

roasted meat platter with horseradish and honey mustard dressing

½ head red-leaf lettuce

350g (12oz) sliced lean deli roast beef

350g (12oz) sliced roast turkey breast

350g (12oz) lean sliced ham (no honey-baked or glazed)

50ml (2fl oz) reduced-fat mayonnaise

275ml (10fl oz) non-fat natural yoghurt

1½ tablespoons horseradish

15g (½oz) snipped chives

1½ tablespoons honey-flavoured mustard

32 slices thin-sliced rye bread (or 16 slices medium-sliced rye bread)

To prepare the meat platter, line a serving platter with lettuce leaves. Place meat in radiating rows from the centre of the platter to the edge, folding the slices in half and overlapping them. The folded edge should show.

To prepare the horseradish sauce, mix the mayonnaise, 115ml (4fl oz) yoghurt, horseradish and chives together and place in a small bowl. Serve with meat platter.

To prepare the Honey Mustard Dressing, mix the remaining yoghurt and honey-flavoured mustard together and place in a small bowl. Serve with the meat platter.

Place bread in a basket near the meat for people to make their own sandwiches.

Makes 8 servings.

Per serving: 453 calories, 39.1 grams protein, 43.8 grams carbohydrate, 12.3 grams fat (2.9 saturated), 87 milligrams cholesterol, 1091 milligrams sodium, 2.1 grams fibre

tomato platter

2 large red tomatoes
2 large yellow tomatoes
1–2 tablespoons Honey Mustard
  Dressing from the Roasted
  Meat Platter
1 bunch watercress, for garnish

Slice tomatoes and alternate slices on a serving platter. Drizzle 1–2 tablespoons Honey Mustard Sauce over. Place sprigs of watercress on the side for a garnish. Makes
Makes 8 servings.

Per serving: 46 calories, 2.4 grams protein, 7.6 grams carbohydrate, 0.4 grams fat (0 saturated), 1.0 milligrams cholesterol, 29 milligrams sodium, 0 grams fibre

pasta salad

50ml (2fl oz) reduced-fat
    mayonnaise
2 tablespoons freshly squeezed
    lemon juice
15g (1/2oz) snipped fresh dill
225g (8oz) uncooked wholemeal
    penne or other wholemeal
    short-cut pasta
150g (5oz) small broccoli florets
1 medium cucumber, peeled,
    seeded and cubed
2 medium red peppers, cubed
Salt and freshly ground black
    pepper to taste

Place a large saucepan with 2–3 litres (4–5 pints) water to boil. Mix mayonnaise, lemon juice and dill together in a large serving bowl. Add pasta to boiling water and cook for 5 minutes. Add broccoli and continue to cook for 4 minutes or until pasta is cooked but still firm. Drain and add to serving bowl. Add cucumber, red pepper and salt and pepper to taste.
Makes 8 servings.

Per serving: 123 calories, 4.7 grams protein,
21.4 grams carbohydrate, 3.0 grams fat
(0.6 saturated), 3 milligrams cholesterol, 66 milligrams
sodium, 3.3 grams fibre

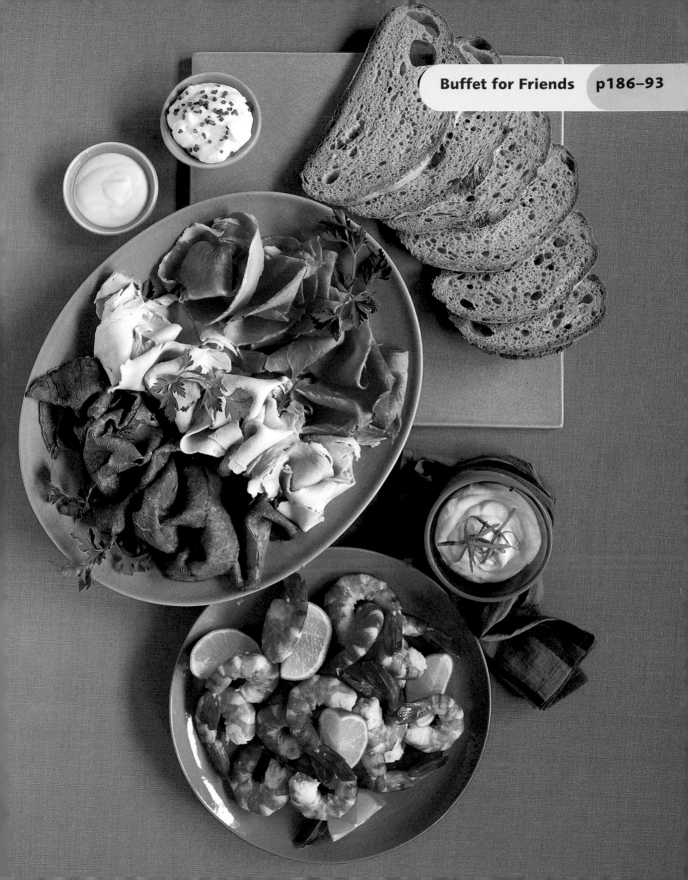

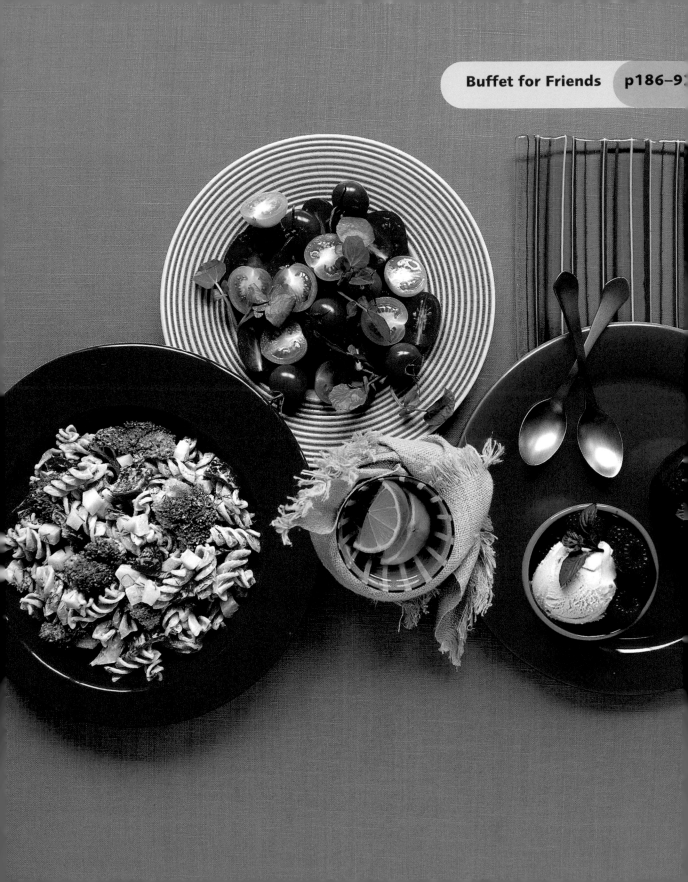

frozen yoghurt berry cup

900ml (32fl oz) low-fat, frozen strawberry yoghurt
1.1kg (2¹/₂lb) fresh raspberries

Spoon yoghurt into 8 dessert bowls and sprinkle berries on top.
Makes 8 servings.

Per serving: 151 calories, 3.6 grams protein, 27.1 grams carbohydrate, 3.4 grams fat (1.5 saturated), 10 milligrams cholesterol, 80 milligrams sodium, 2.9 grams fibre

helpful hints

● *Any fresh berries can be used.*

● *The frozen yoghurt can be spooned into dessert bowls and placed in the freezer in the morning. They only need to be removed and sprinkled with berries just before serving. They will also hold for about 30 minutes out of the freezer this way.*

barbecue
party

barbecue party

The meal fits the nutritional guidelines for the Right Carbs phase.

   'Let's have a barbecue' is an invitation that brings smiles to everyone. Grilled food is popular year-round and the idea of cooking outside brings sunny thoughts to most of us, even in the winter months.

Most barbecued foods are coated with sugary sauces that have a lot of carbs. This simple barbecue party captures the flavours of the grill without the carbohydrates.

It's easiest to serve this meal buffet-style.

Menu

Spicy Tuna Spread

No-Fuss Salad Bar

Lime Barbecued Chicken with Black Bean Sauce

Green Bean and Orzo Salad

Melon with Marinated Strawberries

Countdown

Two days ahead

● Shop for ingredients.

One day ahead

● Make Spicy Tuna Spread.

● Make black bean sauce for chicken. Cover and refrigerate.

● Prepare and blanch onion and red pepper for chicken recipe. Cover and refrigerate.

● Make strawberry sauce and place in a bowl. Cover and refrigerate.

Morning of the party

● Place ingredients for salad bar in attractive bowls. Cover and refrigerate.

● Make Green Bean and Orzo Salad. Wrap and refrigerate.

● Cut melon into slices and place in bowl. Cover and refrigerate.

● Cut cucumber slices for tuna spread. Wrap and refrigerate.

One hour before guests arrive

● Marinate chicken, covered, in refrigerator.

● Light barbecue, if using charcoal.

● Remove tuna spread, black bean sauce, red pepper and onion, orzo salad and strawberry sauce from the refrigerator.

● Arrange melon on individual dessert plates. Cover with clingfilm and set aside.

● Set up salad bar on buffet table.

shopping list

Buy 2 days ahead of party

FRUIT AND VEG
1 bunch basil leaves
1 small bunch parsley
1 small bunch coriander
2 medium cucumbers
*2 bags washed, ready-to-
    eat lettuce*
*1 bag grated, washed,
    ready-to-eat carrots*
*2 bags shredded, washed,
    ready-to-eat red
    cabbage*
*2 bags washed, ready-to-
    eat celery sticks*
2 red peppers
*900g (2lb) fresh green
    beans*
*1kg (2½lb) cherry
    tomatoes*
3 limes
2 lemons
1 honeydew melon
*1.1kg (2½lb) fresh
    strawberries*
DAIRY
*1 small piece Parmesan
    cheese (25g/1oz
    needed for Parmesan
    curls)*
MEAT
*8 x 175g (6oz) boneless
    skinless chicken breasts*

Fifteen minutes before guests arrive

● *Place black bean sauce in a saucepan over low heat to heat through.*

● *Spread tuna on cucumber slices and place on serving platter.*

● *Pre-heat gas barbecue.*

● *While guests are having drinks and hors d'oeuvres, grill chicken and place on platter in low oven to keep warm.*

To serve meal

● *Spoon half the black bean sauce on to a serving platter, place chicken on top and sprinkle with blanched onion and red pepper. Serve the remaining sauce in a bowl*

next to the chicken platter. Place on buffet table.

● *Place orzo salad on buffet table.*

To serve dessert

● *Pre-heat oven and place biscuits in oven while main dishes are being cleared.*

● *Spoon strawberry sauce over melon and place biscuits on side.*

spicy tuna spread

8 stoned green or black olives

175g (6oz) tin tuna packed in
water

2 tablespoons mayonnaise

3 tablespoons horseradish

15g (1/2oz) fresh basil leaves,
washed and dried

2 medium cucumbers, peeled and
sliced on the diagonal

Place olives, tuna, mayonnaise, horseradish and
basil in a food processor and process until
smooth. Taste for seasoning, adding more
horseradish if necessary. Just before serving,
spread on cucumber slices, and place on
serving platter.

Makes 8 servings.

Per serving: 49 calories, 6.3 grams protein, 3.8 grams
carbohydrate, 1.3 grams fat (0.1 saturated),
9 milligrams cholesterol, 199 milligrams sodium,
0.6 grams fibre

shopping list(cont)

GROCERY

1 small container stoned
green or black olives
(8 olives needed)

1 small jar horseradish

1 small packet orzo

1 small container orange juice

1 small packet icing sugar

1 packet almond-flavoured or
other biscuits

STAPLES

175g (6oz) tin tuna packed in
water

Red onion

Garlic

Cayenne pepper

Mayonnaise

No-sugar-added salad
dressings

Tinned black beans
(450g/16oz needed)

Olive oil

Balsamic vinegar

Salt

Black peppercorns

no-fuss salad bar

A colourful salad bar makes a pretty display and is easy to assemble. Here are some tips on how you can put one together without any washing or cutting. Buy a selection of these items from your supermarket: pre-washed lettuce, grated carrots, sliced red cabbage, celery sticks.

2 bags washed, ready-to-eat lettuce
1 bag grated carrots
2 bags shredded red cabbage
2 bags celery sticks
1kg (2¹/₂lb) cherry tomatoes
8 tablespoons no-sugar-added salad dressing

All you need to do is open the bags and place the vegetables in attractive bowls. Add a bowl of rinsed cherry tomatoes. I have given you guidelines, but you can choose whatever vegetables you like. The secret is to make a colourful display. I like to use different sizes and shapes of bowls for the vegetables and dressing. For a party it's nice to fill bowls with the dressings. For nutritional values, plan for 1 tablespoon dressing per person.

Buy 2 different types of dressings. Look for dressings that have no sugar added and are made with olive or rapeseed oil.

Per serving: 201 calories, 15G protein, 12G carbohydrate, 11G fat (3G saturated), 426MG cholestorol, 511MG sodium, 3G fibre

lime-barbecued chicken with black bean sauce

115ml (4fl oz) fresh lime juice

225ml (8fl oz) olive oil

1 teaspoon cayenne pepper

4 garlic cloves, crushed

8 x 175g (6oz) boneless, skinless chicken breasts

50g (2oz) chopped red onion

2 red peppers, diced

50ml (2fl oz) balsamic vinegar

115ml (4fl oz) orange juice

450g(16oz) drained and rinsed cooked tinnned black beans

Salt and freshly ground black pepper

Several sprigs fresh coriander or parsley, for garnish

To prepare the chicken, mix lime juice, oil, cayenne pepper and 2 cloves crushed garlic together and pour into plastic bag or bowl. Add the chicken breasts and marinate overnight or about 8 hours. Remove from refrigerator, drain, and bring to room temperature. Seal the juices in the chicken by browning each piece on both sides, about 2 minutes per side. Move chicken to a cooler area of barbecue to finish cooking without burning, about 5 minutes.

To prepare for Black Bean Sauce, mix vinegar, orange juice, remaining 2 cloves garlic, and black beans together and purée in a blender or food processor. Add salt and pepper to taste. Warm in a microwave or in a saucepan. To blanch the onion and red pepper, bring a pot of water to the boil and add the onion and red pepper. As soon as the water returns to the boil, drain and rinse under cold water. Or place in a microwave-safe bowl and microwave on high for 3 minutes.

To serve, spoon a little Black Bean Sauce on a serving platter and place the chicken over the sauce. Sprinkle the top with the onion and red pepper. Garnish the platter with coriander or parsley. Serve the remaining sauce on the side. *Makes 2 servings.*

Per serving: 353 calories, 54.0 grams protein, 15.2 grams carbohydrate, 9.3 grams fat (1.9 saturated), 132 milligrams cholesterol, 117 milligrams sodium, 1.8 grams fibre

helpful hints

● *Make sure the grill bars on your barbecue are clean. Spray with vegetable oil spray. If using charcoal, heat the barbecue for about 45 minutes before use or 15 minutes if using gas. The coals should be glowing and the bars hot.*

● *If you do not have a barbecue, then brown the chicken in a very hot sauté pan.*

● *An easy way to marinate the chicken is to place it and the marinade in a self-seal plastic bag. It takes up less space in the refrigerator than a bowl and can be easily flipped over to make sure all sides of the chicken are marinated.*

green bean and orzo salad

225g (8oz) orzo

900g (2lb) fresh green beans, trimmed and cut into 2.5cm (1in) pieces

50ml (2fl oz) olive oil and vinegar dressing

Salt and freshly ground black pepper

25g (1oz) Parmesan cheese

Bring a large saucepan with 3–4 litres (5–7 pints) of water to the boil over high heat. Add the orzo and boil for 5 minutes. Add the beans and continue to boil for 5 minutes more. Drain. Place in a serving bowl and drizzle the dressing on top and toss well. Add salt and pepper to taste. Make Parmesan curls by thinly slicing the Parmesan with a potato peeler. Place the curls on top of the salad.

Makes 8servings.

Per serving: 224 calories, 7.2 grams protein, 30.0 grams carbohydrate, 10.1grams fat (2.6 saturated), 3 milligrams cholesterol, 108 milligrams sodium, 3.4 grams fibre

melon with marinated strawberries

1 honeydew melon, sliced

1.1kg (2½lb) fresh strawberries

3 tablespoons icing sugar, sifted

2 tablespoons freshly squeezed
   lemon juice

8 almond-flavoured or other
   bought biscuits

Wash, hull and slice strawberries. Blend in sugar and lemon juice. Leave to marinate for 3–4 hours.

Place 2 slices melon on each dessert plate and spoon strawberry sauce on top. Serve 1 biscuit on the side of each plate.

Makes 8 servings.

Per serving: 126 calories, 2.3 grams protein,
30.2 grams carbohydrate, 1 gram fat (0 saturated),
0 milligrams cholesterol, 16 milligrams sodium,
3.3 grams fibre

index

apples
Cranberry Apple Sauce 161
Pork Chops with Apple Relish
160–161
artichokes
Sausage and Artichoke Frittata 37
asparagus
Braised Asparagus 53
Roasted Asparagus with Red Pepper
178
Aubergine Parmesan with Linguine 79

bacon
BLT Sandwich on Rye 104
Bacon and Cheese Crêpes 31
Barbecue Party 194–201
beans
Black Bean Soup with Rice 138
Chicken with Black Bean Salsa 86–87
French Green Beans 155
Lime Barbecued Chicken with Black
Bean Sauce 199
Mexican Sopes 122–123
Peasant Country Soup 132
Three Bean Salad 185
beef
Beef Teriyaki with Chinese Noodles
134
Blue Cheese and Beef Pasta Salad 106
Garlic-Stuffed Steak 144–145
Mock Hungarian Goulash 139
Roast Beef and Cucumber Slices 62
Spiced Cowboy Steak 149
Steak in Port Wine 154–155
Berry Cups with Almond Sauce 179
beverages
Ginger-Cranberry Smoothie with
Smoked Ham and Cheese 64
Black Bean Soup with Rice 138
BLT Sandwich on Rye 104
Blue Cheese and Beef Pasta Salad 106
blueprints 12
bran cereal 61, 64, 66, 98, 100
breads

BLT Sandwich on Rye 104
Bruschetta 175
Danish Prawn Smorrebrod 109
Grilled Halibut Sandwich 184
Herb Cheese Toast and Salad 132
Italian Croque Monsieur 69
Mediterranean Scramble on Toast 99
Monte Cristo Sandwich 100
Smoked Salmon Sandwich 96
broccoli
Toasted Almond Broccoli 55
Brown Rice with Toasted Pinenuts 177
Bruschetta 175
Buffet for Friends 186–193

cabbage
Sweet and Sour Cabbage 153
Cajun Prawn Salad 7
Casual Soup Supper 180–185
celery
Chicken with Dill Mustard 40
Smoked Salmon-Stuffed Celery 36
cereal, bran 61, 64, 66, 98, 100
cheese
Bacon and Cheese Crêpes 31
Blue Cheese and Beef Pasta Salad 106
Cheese and Chicken Bundles 41
Bacon and Cheese Crêpes 31
Greek Prawns with Feta Cheese 127
Herb Cheese Toast and Salad 132
Italian Croque Monsieur 69
Microwave Marinara Scramble 35
Monte Cristo Sandwich 100
Parmesan Courgettes 147
Parmesan Sole 135
Strawberry Splash with Cottage
Cheese-Stuffed Chicory 97
String Beans with Crumbled
Gorgonzola 170
Turkey Salsa Roll 34
chicken
Cheese and Chicken Bundles 41
Chicken and Walnuts in Lettuce Puffs
152–153

Chicken Burgers with Warm
Mushroom Salad 50
Chinese Chicken Salad 75
Chicken Creole 136–137
Chicken Tonnato 168
Chicken with Black Bean Salsa 86–87
Chicken with Dill Mustard 40
Crunchy Oriental Chicken Salad 44
Dijon Chicken with Crunchy
Couscous 143
Hawaiian Chicken with Pineapple
Caesar Salad 120–121
Indian-Spiced Chicken 157
Lime Barbecued Chicken with Black
Bean Sauce 199
Mexican Sopes 122–123
Mulligatawny Soup 103
Nutty Chicken Minestrone 42
Peasant Country Soup 132
Rainbow Tomato Plate 73
Roast Chicken Vegetable Soup 72
Savoury Sage Chicken 129
Tuscan Chicken 54
chicory
Chicory and Orange Salad with Swiss
Turkey 107
Strawberry Splash with Cottage
Cheese-Stuffed Chicory 97
Red Pepper and Chicory Salad 47
chocolate
White Chocolate Whip 171
coleslaw
Crab Cakes and Slaw 51
cooking tips 21
countdown 12
courgettes
Courgette Gratin 49
Parmesan Courgettes 147

crab
Crab Cakes and Slaw 51
Crab Gratin 45
Vietnamese Crab Soup 70
Creamy Wild Mushroom Soup 183

crêpes and pancakes
 Bacon and Cheese Crêpes 31
Crispy Cod with Ratatouille 77–78
cucumber
 Roast Beef and Cucumber Slices 62

Danish Prawn Smorrebrod 109
deli department 15
desserts
 Berry Cups with Almond Sauce 179
 Cranberry Apple Sauce 161
 Frozen Yoghurt Berry Cup 193
 Lemon Chiffon 159
 Mango Fool 185
 Melon with Marinated Strawberries 201
 Pears with Raspberry Coulis 151
 White Chocolate Whip 171
Dijon Chicken with Crunchy Couscous 143
dining out 23–24
Dinner Party for Eight 172–179
Dr. Atkins' New Diet Revolution 16

eating out 23–24
eggs
 Ham and Pepper Frittata 95
 Ham-Baked Egg 65
 Italian Omelette 66
 Microwave Eggs Parmesan 32
 Microwave Marinara Scramble 35
 Microwave Portobello Scramble 98
 Monte Cristo Sandwich 100
 Mushroom, Turkey and Tarragon Omelette 33
 New Orleans Prawn Roll 67
 Provençal Omelette 101
 Sausage and Artichoke Frittata 37
 Sausage Scramble 63
electric cooking 21
entertaining 162–201
equipment 20–21

fish
 Crispy Cod with Ratatouille 77–78
 Five-Spice Tuna Tataki 84–85
 Grilled Halibut Sandwich 184
 Horseradish-Crusted Salmon Salad 74
 Mahi Mahi Satay with Thai Peanut Sauce 112–113
 Mediterranean Baked Fish 48
 Pan-Seared Tuna with Mango Salsa 158–159
 Parmesan Sole 135

 Roasted Pepper and Olive Snapper 118–119
 Roasted Salmon and Herb Sauce 53
 Smoked Salmon Sandwich 96
 Smoked Salmon-Stuffed Celery 36
 Spanish Tuna-Stuffed Tomatoes 43
 Spicy Tuna Spread 197
 Swordfish in Spanish Sofrito Sauce 131
 Whisky-Soused Salmon 116–117
 see also cod, tuna etc
Five-Spice Tuna Tataki 84–85
flexibility 12
food processors 20
Frozen Yoghurt Berry Cup 193
fruits
 Cranberry Apple Sauce 161
 Frozen Yoghurt Berry Cup 193
 Mango Fool 185
 Melon with Marinated Strawberries 201
 see also individual fruits

Garden Crudités and Dips 167
Garlic-Stuffed Steak 144–145
Ginger-Cranberry Smoothie with Smoked Ham and Cheese 64
grains
 Dijon Chicken with Crunchy Couscous 143
 Green Bean and Orzo Salad 200
 Lentil and Rice Salad 169
 Toasted Walnut Lentils 161
Greek Prawns with Feta Cheese 127
Green Bean and Orzo Salad 200
Grilled Halibut Sandwich 184
Guinea Fowl in Red Wine 176

ham
 Ham and Pepper Frittata 95
 Ham-Baked Egg 65
 Italian Croque Monsieur 69
 Microwave Marinara Scramble 35
 Veal Saltimbocca 146–147
Hawaiian Chicken with Pineapple Caesar Salad 120–121
helpful hints 12, 21–22
herbs
 Herb Cheese Toast and Salad 132
 Mushroom, Turkey and Tarragon Omelette 33
 Provençal Omelette 101
 Roasted Salmon and Herb Sauce 53
 Savoury Sage Chicken 129

 Turkey Gratinée with Basil Linguine 114–115
 Horseradish-Crusted Salmon Salad 74
 Veal Saltimbocca 146–147
Hot Pepper Prawns 47

Indian-Spiced Chicken 157
insulin 27
Italian Croque Monsieur 69
Italian Omelette 66
Italian Supper for Friends 164–171

Jamaican Jerk Pork 128

labels, reading 16–18
Layered Antipasto Salad 105
legumes. *See* beans
lentils
 Lentil and Rice Salad 169
lettuce
 BLT Sandwich on Rye 104
 Cheese and Chicken Bundles 41
 Chicken and Walnuts in Lettuce Puffs 152–153
 Radicchio, Chicory and Watercress Salad 175
'light', meaning of 16
Lime Barbecued Chicken with Black Bean Sauce 199
'low-fat', meaning of 16

Mahi Mahi Satay with Thai Peanut Sauce 112–113
mango
 Mango Fool 185
 Pan-Seared Tuna with Mango Salsa 158–159
meats
 Roasted Meat Platter with Horseradish and Honey Mustard Dressing 190
 see also chicken, beef etc
Mediterranean Baked Fish 48
Mediterranean Scramble on Toast 99
Mediterranean Snapper with Provençal Salad 150–151
Mediterranean Steak 80–81
melon.
 Melon with Marinated Strawberries 201
Mexican Sopes 122–123
Microwave Eggs Parmesan 32
Microwave Marinara Scramble 35

Microwave Portobello Scramble 98
Mock Hungarian Goulash 139
Monte Cristo Sandwich 100
mozzarella
  Italian Croque Monsieur 69
  Microwave Marinara Scramble 35
Mulligatawny Soup 103
Mushroom and Sausage Soup 108
Mushroom, Turkey and Tarragon
  Omelette
mushrooms
  Chicken Burgers with Warm
  Mushroom Salad 50
  Creamy Wild Mushroom Soup 183
  Microwave Portobello Scramble 98
  Mock Hungarian Goulash 139
  Mushroom and Sausage Soup 108
  Mushroom, Turkey and Tarragon
  Omelette 33
  Peasant Country Soup 132
  Pork Escalopes with Spinach and
  Mushrooms 52
  Sicilian Baked Mushrooms and
  Sausage 39

New Orleans Prawn Roll 67
No-Fuss Salad Bar 198
noodles. See pasta
nuts
  Berry Cups with Almond Sauce 179
  Brown Rice with Toasted Pinenuts 177
  Cheese and Chicken Bundles 41
  Chicken and Walnuts in Lettuce Puffs
  152–153
  Mahi Mahi Satay with Thai Peanut
  Sauce 112–113
  Nutty Chicken Minestrone 42
  Rainbow Tomato Plate 73
  Toasted Almond Broccoli 55
  Toasted Walnut Lentils 161

oatmeal 63, 65, 67, 99, 101
omelettes
  Ham and Pepper Frittata 95
  Italian Omelette 66
  Mushroom, Turkey and Tarragon
  Omelette 33
  Provençal Omelette 101
  Sausage and Artichoke Frittata 37
olives
  Mediterranean Scramble on Toast 99
  Roasted Pepper and Olive Snapper
  118–119
pancakes. See crêpes and pancakes

Pan-Seared Tuna with Mango Salsa
  158–159
Parmesan Sole 135
pasta
  Aubergine Parmesan with Linguine 79
  Blue Cheese and Beef Pasta Salad 106
  Pasta Salad 192
  Beef Teriyaki with Chinese Noodles
  134
  Turkey Gratinée with Basil Linguine
  114–115
pears
  Pears with Raspberry Coulis 151
Peasant Country Soup 132
peppers
  Roasted Asparagus with Red Pepper
  178
  Roasted Pepper and Olive Snapper
  118–119
  Red Pepper and Chicory Salad 47
pork
  Jamaican Jerk Pork 128
  Pork Chops with Apple Relish
  160–161
  Pork Escalopes with Spinach and
  Mushrooms 52
  Roast Pork with Strawberry Salsa 111
portion sizes 24
poultry
  Guinea Fowl in Red Wine 176
  see also chicken; turkey
prawns
  Cajun Prawn Salad 71
  Danish Prawn Smorrebrod 109
  Greek Prawns with Feta Cheese 127
  Hot Pepper Prawns 47
  New Orleans Prawn Roll 67
  Prawns in Lime-Mustard Sauce 189
Protein Power 10
Provençal Omelette 101

Quick Cooking Tips 21–22
Quick Start phase 28–54
  14-Day Meal Plan 28–29
  Breakfasts 30–37
  Dinners 46–54
  Lunches 38–45
  Super Speed Suppers 126–129
  Weekend Meals 142–147

Radicchio, Chicory and Watercress Salad
  175
Rainbow Tomato Plate 73
raspberries

Pears with Raspberry Coulis 151
'reduced-fat', meaning of 16
restaurants 23–24
rice
  Black Bean Soup with Rice 138
  Brown Rice 155
  Brown Rice with Toasted Pinenuts 177
  Lentil and Rice Salad 169
  Rice and Spinach Pilaf 157
  Saffron Pilaf 159
  Yellow Rice 131
Right Carb phase 90–123
  14-Day Meal Plan 92–93
  Breakfasts 94–101
  Dinners 110–123
  Lunches 102–109
  Super Speed Suppers 134–139
  Weekend Meals 156–161
Roast Beef and Cucumber Slices 62
Roast Chicken Vegetable Soup 72
Roast Pork with Strawberry Salsa 111
Roasted Asparagus with Red Pepper 178
Roasted Meat Platter with Horseradish
  and Honey Mustard Dressing 190
Roasted Pepper and Olive Snapper
  118–119
Roasted Salmon and Herb Sauce 53

salads
  Blue Cheese and Beef Pasta Salad 106
  Cajun Prawn Salad 71
  Chicken Burgers with Warm
  Mushroom Salad 50
  Chinese Chicken Salad 75
  Crunchy Oriental Chicken Salad 44
  Green Bean and Orzo Salad 200
  Hawaiian Chicken with Pineapple
  Caesar Salad 120–121
  Herb Cheese Toast and Salad 132
  Horseradish-Crusted Salmon Salad 74
  Italian Salad 147
  Layered Antipasto Salad 105
  Lentil and Rice Salad 169
  No-Fuss Salad Bar 198
  Provençal Salad 150
  Radicchio, Chicory and Watercress
  Salad 175
  Red Pepper and Chicory Salad 47
  Three Bean Salad 185
salmon
  Horseradish-Crusted Salmon Salad 74
  Roasted Salmon and Herb Sauce 53
  Smoked Salmon Sandwich 96
  Smoked Salmon-Stuffed Celery 36
  Whisky-Soused Salmon 116–117

salsa
Chicken with Black Bean Salsa 86–87
Pan-Seared Tuna with Mango Salsa
158–159
Roast Pork with Strawberry Salsa 111
Turkey Salsa Roll 34
sandwiches
BLT Sandwich on Rye 104
Danish Prawn Smorrebrod 109
Grilled Halibut Sandwich 184
Italian Croque Monsieur 69
Monte Cristo Sandwich 100
Smoked Salmon Sandwich 96
sauces
Cranberry Apple Sauce 161Roasted
Salmon and Herb Sauce 53
Swordfish in Spanish Sofrito Sauce
131
sausage
Mushroom and Sausage Soup 108
Sausage and Artichoke Frittata 37
Sausage Scramble 63
Sicilian Baked Mushrooms and
Sausage 39
Savoury Sage Chicken 129
seafood
Cajun Prawn Salad 71
Danish Prawn Smorrebrod 109
Greek Prawns with Feta Cheese 127
Hot Pepper Prawns 47
New Orleans Prawn Roll 67
Vietnamese Crab Soup 70
shellfish. See seafood
shopping
shopping 14
shopping Guidelines 17–18
smart shopping 9–10
supermarket shopping 15–16
Sicilian Baked Mushrooms and Sausage
39
slices, weight of 22

Smoked Salmon Sandwich 96
Smoked Salmon-Stuffed Celery 36
smoothies
Ginger-Cranberry Smoothie with
Smoked Ham and Cheese 64
Strawberry Splash with Cottage
Cheese-Stuffed Chicory 97
snack ideas 25
sole
Parmesan Sole 135
soups
Black Bean Soup with Rice 138
Creamy Wild Mushroom Soup 183
Mulligatawny Soup 103

Mushroom and Sausage Soup 108
Nutty Chicken Minestrone 42
Peasant Country Soup 132
Roast Chicken Vegetable Soup 72
Vietnamese Crab Soup 70
Spanish Tuna-Stuffed Tomatoes 43
Spiced Cowboy Steak 149
Spicy Tuna Spread 197
spinach
Microwave Marinara Scramble 35
Pork Escalopes with Spinach and
Mushrooms 52
Rice and Spinach Pilaf 157
staples 19–20
Steak in Port Wine 154–155
Stir-Fried Veal 82–83
strawberries
Melon with Marinated Strawberries
201
Strawberry Splash with Cottage
Cheese-Stuffed Chicory 97
String Beans with Crumbled Gorgonzola
170
Sugar Busters 10
'sugar-free', meaning of 16
Super Speed Suppers 124–139
supermarket aisles 15–16
supermarket shopping 15–16
Swordfish in Spanish Sofrito Sauce 131

The Carbohydrate Addict's Diet 10
Three Bean Salad 185
tips for eating out 23
tomatoes
BLT Sandwich on Rye 104
Bruschetta 175
Chicken Creole 136–137
Tomato Frittata 61
Tomato Platter 191
Chicken Creole 136–137
Rainbow Tomato Plate 73
Spanish Tuna-Stuffed Tomatoes 43
tortillas
Mexican Sopes 122–123
tuna
Chicken Tonnato 168
Five-Spice Tuna Tataki 84–85
Pan-Seared Tuna with Mango Salsa
158–159
Spanish Tuna-Stuffed Tomatoes 43
Spicy Tuna Spread 197
turkey
Turkey Gratinée with Basil Linguine
114–115
Turkey Salsa Roll 34

Monte Cristo Sandwich 100
Mushroom, Turkey and Tarragon
Omelette 33
Tuscan Chicken 54

veal
Veal Piccata 88–89
Veal Saltimbocca 146–147
Stir-Fried Veal 82–83
vegetables
Aubergine Parmesan with Linguine 79
Braised Asparagas 53
Courgette Gratin 49
French Green Beans 155
Garden Crudités and Dips 167
Green Bean and Orzo Salad 200
Parmesan Courgettes 147
Roasted Asparagus with Red Pepper
178
Smoked Salmon-Stuffed Celery 36
String Beans with Crumbled
Gorgonzola 170
Sweet and Sour Cabbage 153
Toasted Almond Broccoli 55
Vietnamese Crab Soup 70

Weekends 140–161
Which Carb phase 56–89
14-Day Meal Plan 58–59
Breakfasts 60–67
Dinners 76–89
Lunches 68–75
Super Speed Suppers 130–134
Weekend Meals 148–155
Whisky-Soused Salmon 116–117
White Chocolate Whip 171

yoghurt
Frozen Yoghurt Berry Cup 193
Ginger-Cranberry Smoothie 64

Zone, The 10

notes

acknowledgments

This book could not have been written without the patience and help of my husband, Harold. From the minute his cardiologist suggested he adopt a low-carbohydrate lifestyle seven years ago, he has helped me to create and test these recipes. Many thanks and much love.

Once again my assistant, Jackie Murrill, spent hours helping me test the recipes and always with a smile. Thank you, Jackie, for your friendship and help.

At Bay Books, James Connolly, Publisher, and Bill Schwartz, CEO, have worked endlessly and with great enthusiasm to bring this book to print. Thank you both for helping to bring my words to life. Thanks also to my editor Floyd Yearout. You've been a delight to work with.

Lisa Ekus has been my trusted friend for many years and as my agent was a wonderful help in bringing my ideas to the page. Many thanks, Lisa.

I'd also like to thank my family who have always supported my projects and encouraged me every step of the way: my son James, his wife, Patty, and their sons, Zachary and Jacob, who helped taste these recipes; my son Charles and his wife, Lori, who tested recipes via e-mail; my son John, his wife, Jill, and their children, Jeffrey and Joanna, who cheered me on; my sister Roberta and brother-in-law Robert who helped to edit my thoughts and words.

Thanks go to Kathy Martin, my editor at the *Miami Herald*, who has been a friend and booster for my columns and books.

Thank you to Joseph Cooper, Radio Manager for WLRN National Public Radio for South Florida, who has helped and encouraged me with my 'Food News and Views' segment on his programme, *Topical Currents*.

Thank you to my dear friends, Shep and Bernita King, for letting us take over their kitchen for the original cover photograph.

I'd like to thank the many readers who correspond with me from all over the U.S. to say how much they enjoy the recipes and how much better they feel. This kind of encouragement makes the lonely time in front of the computer worthwhile.

Most important, I'd like to thank all of you who read this book and prepare the meals. I hope you enjoy them and reap the benefits as much as I've enjoyed creating the recipes and watching the wonderful results.